NEUROSCIENCE RESEARCH PROGRESS

ADHD - A TRANSPARENT IMPAIRMENT, CLINICAL, DAILY-LIFE AND RESEARCH ASPECTS IN DIVERSE POPULATIONS

NEUROSCIENCE RESEARCH PROGRESS

Additional books in this series can be found on Nova's website
under the Series tab.

Additional e-books in this series can be found on Nova's website
under the e-book tab.

NEUROSCIENCE RESEARCH PROGRESS

ADHD - A TRANSPARENT IMPAIRMENT, CLINICAL, DAILY-LIFE AND RESEARCH ASPECTS IN DIVERSE POPULATIONS

ITAI BERGER, M.D.
AND
ADINA MAEIR, PH.D.
EDITORS

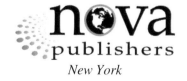
nova
publishers
New York

For permission to use material from this book please contact us:
Telephone 631-231-7269; Fax 631-231-8175
Web Site: http://www.novapublishers.com

NOTICE TO THE READER

The Publisher has taken reasonable care in the preparation of this book, but makes no expressed or implied warranty of any kind and assumes no responsibility for any errors or omissions. No liability is assumed for incidental or consequential damages in connection with or arising out of information contained in this book. The Publisher shall not be liable for any special, consequential, or exemplary damages resulting, in whole or in part, from the readers' use of, or reliance upon, this material. Any parts of this book based on government reports are so indicated and copyright is claimed for those parts to the extent applicable to compilations of such works.

Independent verification should be sought for any data, advice or recommendations contained in this book. In addition, no responsibility is assumed by the publisher for any injury and/or damage to persons or property arising from any methods, products, instructions, ideas or otherwise contained in this publication.

This publication is designed to provide accurate and authoritative information with regard to the subject matter covered herein. It is sold with the clear understanding that the Publisher is not engaged in rendering legal or any other professional services. If legal or any other expert assistance is required, the services of a competent person should be sought. FROM A DECLARATION OF PARTICIPANTS JOINTLY ADOPTED BY A COMMITTEE OF THE AMERICAN BAR ASSOCIATION AND A COMMITTEE OF PUBLISHERS.

Additional color graphics may be available in the e-book version of this book.

Library of Congress Cataloging-in-Publication Data

ISBN: 978-1-63321-047-9

Library of Congress Control Number: 2014939922

Published by Nova Science Publishers, Inc. † New York

CONTENTS

PREFACE

Even an experienced professional might minimize the prevalence of Attention Deficit Hyperactivity Disorder (ADHD) among certain groups of patients. Decreased attention, hyperactivity, and impulsivity are sensitive but non-specific behavioral patterns, frequently reported in a wide range of children and adults with different disorders. Therefore, the existence of ADHD might become "transparent" for both the patients and the professionals. Such transparency might lead to a non-accurate diagnosis, harm the treatment aspects and has potential non beneficial prognostic aspects.

Among children and adults with mental retardation, autistic spectrum disorders, or drug abuse, as well as among gifted children, children with sensory modulation disorders, and children who were born IUGR, the diagnosis of ADHD might be very challenging. It seems that among these "double-diagnosis" populations there is a higher prevalence of patients with ADHD than in the general population, yet the exact prevalence, diagnostic difficulties and treatment methods have not been clearly estimated or established. It also seems that the percentage of ADHD among adolescent and children with chronic illness is still underestimated, since its clinical characteristics tend to be different. During the last years there are growing numbers of publications in this field. But due to the wide range of interested professionals, these studies are published in a wide range of journals usually missing some of their "target" populations. There is a lack of volumes gathering relevant data for a broad range of interested professionals from different specialties.

The objective of this book is to serve as a useful tool for a wide range of professionals with special interest in the unusual aspects of ADHD in order to increase their knowledge, sensitivity and treatment methods among our "transparent" patients.

In: ADHD
Editors: Itai Berger and Adina Maeir

ISBN: 978-1-63321-047-9
© 2014 Nova Science Publishers, Inc.

Chapter 1

IT TAKES A VILLAGE TO CARE FOR ATTENTION-DEFICIT/HYPERACTIVITY DISORDER: IMPROVING MANAGEMENT COLLABORATION BETWEEN TERTIARY CARE CENTERS AND THE COMMUNITY

Ortal Slobodin, Ph.D. and Itai Berger, M.D. [*]
The Neuro-Cognitive Center, Pediatric Division,
Hadassah-Hebrew University Medical Center, Jerusalem, Israel

ABSTRACT

Attention-deficit/hyperactivity disorder (ADHD) is the most common childhood neuro-developmental complaint presenting to clinicians in primary care. ADHD is a chronic, serious cognitive and behavior disorder, which is characterized by heterogeneity, ambiguity, and high comorbidity, and thus cannot lend itself to a universal treatment package. Because no single intervention is optimally effective, the literature supports a multimodal approach which would ideally have available comprehensive services, including medical, mental health, education, social services, and community resources. In 2000, the American Academy of Pediatrics developed evidence based clinical practice guidelines for the diagnosis and evaluation of school-aged children with ADHD in primary care settings. However, research on the implementation of the AAP guidelines by primary care practitioners revealed that they encounter multiple barriers in the management of ADHD, including limited knowledge and experience in managing ADHD, lack of time, financial constraints, and poor communication with education professionals and mental health clinicians. This chapter reviews the aims and challenges in providing adequate care for children with ADHD and their families in primary care settings. Further, an alternative, multidisciplinary care model is proposed, which highlights the importance of specialized services provided at a tertiary care level. Ideally, this model should adopt principles of care for chronic conditions, such as family-centered

[*] Correspondence: Itai Berger, MD. The Neuro-Cognitive Center, Pediatric Division, Hadassah-Hebrew University Medical Center, P.O. Box 24035, Mount Scopus Campus, Jerusalem, Israel, E-mail: itberg@hadassah.org.il.

system of care, shared decision-making and ongoing education to primary care providers. Such a solution would allow sharing resources and expertise between service providers and thus could ensure not only a professional, shortened process of diagnosis and treatment but also a patient-centered intervention that would take into account individuals' needs and preferences.

INTRODUCTION

Attention-deficit/hyperactivity disorder (ADHD) is the most common childhood neuro-developmental complaint presenting to clinicians in primary care [1-3]. ADHD affects 4% to 12% of United States children, depending on diagnostic tools [4, 5], diagnostic criteria, [6, 7], and studied samples [8]. Despite such a high prevalence, the heterogeneous, complex manifestation of ADHD leads to considerable variation in the diagnosis and treatment of this disorder. ADHD symptoms (i.e., hyperactivity, inattention, and impulsivity) lie on a spectrum from normal childhood behavior to substantial disorder and are associated with a maturational delay [9-13]. Thus, the diagnosis of ADHD is difficult to make in younger pre-school children, as many normal preschool children are more hyperactive and impulsive and have a shorter attention span than a majority of the older children [14]. Furthermore, ADHD usually co-exists with a variety of medical, developmental, psychiatric, and cognitive conditions which can present very similar symptoms [15, 16]. Among children in primary care settings, it is estimated that 40% have oppositional defiant disorder or conduct disorder and 10% have depressive disorders [17, 18]. The lack of a precise, objective measure of ADHD further contributes to the variability in diagnosis [19, 20]. These factors have raised major concerns among the medical community about over-diagnosis and treatment [21].

THE MANAGEMENT OF ADHD IN PRIMARY CARE PRACTICE

A major venue for the delivery of services to children with ADHD in most European and North-American countries is primary care [2, 22, 23]. In most cases, the professional works in isolation rather than as a part of a multidisciplinary team and when indicated refers the child for further assessment to another professional with complementary skills [24]. Although youths with ADHD constitute up to 50% of the child psychiatry clinic population [25], at least 50% of patients with ADHD are not treated for ADHD by a mental health specialist [2, 26]. This is probably due to a combination of factors, such as the high prevalence of ADHD, families' perceptions of the role of primary care providers, and the limited availability of mental health professionals [5, 27]. The fact that pediatricians are expected to treat large proportions of children and adolescents with ADHD means that they need to be skilled in the diagnosis and treatment of ADHD. However, a growing number of professionals have raised concerns regarding the quality of ADHD diagnosis and treatment in primary care settings [2, 28, 29]. One of the criticisms frequently voiced in the medical literature and popular media is that ADHD management by primary care providers (PCPs) is often limited to psychopharmacological treatments [28, 30, 31]. Although medication therapy is the cornerstone of ADHD treatment and its efficacy is well established, it is mistakenly considered as the sole intervention [28]. Efficacy studies, including the large scale multi-site

MTA study (Multimodal Treatment Study of Children with Attention-Deficit Hyperactivity Disorder), suggest that behavior treatment and parent education are equally important components of successful treatment of ADHD [20, 32-34]. It has also been shown that children with ADHD treated in the community with stimulant medications make gains in academics but remain significantly impaired relative to their peers [35]. Further, stimulants do not address the wide range of interpersonal problems children with ADHD experience [36, 37]. Because most children are treated in the community, primarily by their primary care providers, the apparent lack of relative efficacy of ADHD medication treatment in community settings compared with university settings poses a significant public health concern [38].

In order to address these concerns, the Council on Scientific Affairs (CSA) of the American Medical Association published in 1997 several recommendations for the diagnosis and treatment of ADHD in the community [39]. Among the CSA's recommendation were (a) to encourage physicians to utilize standardized diagnostic criteria in making diagnosis of ADHD (e.g., DSM-IV TR), (b) to increase training about ADHD in medical schools, residency programs, the importance of individualized treatment approaches for children with ADHD, which include psychopharmacology, behavior treatment, psychoeducation, and school-based interventions and (c) to cooperate with schools to improve teachers' recognition of ADHD symptoms to make appropriate recommendations to parents and health-care professionals. One of the recommendations was to create and disseminate practice guidelines for ADHD by specialists to practicing physicians.

Subsequently, in 2000, the American Academy of Pediatrics [40] has affirmed the critical role of primary care providers (PCPs) in the delivery of services to children with ADHD. To emphasize the importance of accurate and evidence based ADHD diagnosis, the AAP, through its Committee on Quality Improvement, has developed an evidence based clinical practice guideline for the diagnosis and evaluation of the school-aged children with ADHD (table 1). The AAP published two sets of ADHD practice guidelines for children aged 6 to 12 years: one for evaluation and the second for management, both are specifically geared toward the general pediatrician and family physician. The AAP assessment guidelines emphasize the importance of collecting parent and teacher standardized rating scales and using the Diagnostic and Statistical Manual of Mental Disorders Fourth Edition (DSM-IV) criteria as the basis for making an ADHD diagnosis. These guidelines highlight the importance of obtaining information from the child, parents, and teachers about ADHD and potential comorbid conditions in conducting an assessment of ADHD. Also, the guidelines emphasize that treatment planning should represent a collaborative effort among the family, school, and health systems and that treatment, including pharmacologic and/or behavioral methods, should be designed to improve specified academic and behavioral targets. These guidelines have been reported in various journals and adopted by other organizations, including the American Academy of Family Physicians and large insurers and managed care organizations [41, 42].

Research on the implementation of the AAP guidelines suggests that although it was generally acknowledged by primary care clinicians and incorporated into their practices, there are many obstacles in systematically following its recommendations [3, 43, 44]. A survey conducted among 1000 primary care pediatricians and family physicians in the United States, revealed that very few practitioners report practices that follow the AAP guideline as a whole, especially concerning the use of DSM criteria and other laboratory and diagnostic tests [43].

Table 1. Summary of the American Academy of Pediatrics Clinical Practice Guideline for Diagnosis and Evaluation of the Child with Attention Deficit Hyperactivity Disorder [40]

		Recommendations
1.		In a child 6–12 years old who presents with inattention, hyperactivity, impulsivity, academic underachievement, or behavior problems, primary care clinicians should initiate an evaluation of ADHD.
2.		The diagnosis of ADHD requires that a child meet Diagnostic and Statistical Manual of Mental Disorders–IV criteria.
3.		The assessment of ADHD requires evidence directly obtained from parents or caregivers regarding the core symptoms of ADHD in various settings, the age of onset, duration of symptoms, and degree of functional impairment.
	3A.	Use of ADHD-specific parent rating scales is a clinical option when evaluating children for ADHD.
	3B.	Use of broadband parent rating scales is not recommended in the diagnosis of children for ADHD, although they may be useful for other purposes.
4.		The assessment of ADHD requires evidence directly obtained from the classroom teacher (or other school professional) regarding the core symptoms of ADHD, the duration of symptoms, the degree of functional impairment, and coexisting conditions. A physician should review any reports from a school-based multidisciplinary evaluation where they exist, which will include assessments from the teacher or other school-based professional.
	4A.	Use of ADHD-specific teacher rating scales is a clinical option when diagnosing children for ADHD.
	4B.	Use of teacher global questionnaires and rating scales is not recommended in the diagnosing of children for ADHD, although they may be useful for other purposes.
5.		Evaluation of the child with ADHD should include assessment for coexisting conditions.
6.		Other diagnostic tests are not routinely indicated to establish the diagnosis of ADHD.

According to this study, fewer than 60% of physicians reported using any formal criteria to diagnose ADHD, and of those, less than one third used DSM criteria. Up to one quarter of the physicians reported the routine use of other diagnostic tests to establish the diagnosis of ADHD. Moreover, one -fifth to one third of physicians do not routinely incorporate teacher and school information into the evaluation process, as the guideline recommends [43].

Studies examining potential barriers in adopting the published guidelines suggest that multiple factors might be involved in the observed discrepancies between primary care practice patterns and the AAP guidelines (table 2). First, many primary care practitioners have limited knowledge regarding the diagnosis and treatment of ADHD, mainly due to a lack of formalized training. Consequently, they may be more likely to under-diagnose [45-47] or over-diagnose ADHD [48] and less likely to recognize coexisting mental health conditions compared to mental health professionals [3, 43]. The study of Chan and co-workers [43] indicated that 10%–25% of physicians did not assess conditions such as tic disorder, language disorder, and oppositional-defiant disorder. Assessment of coexisting conditions is essential for accurate diagnosis because many conditions may mimic or exacerbate ADHD symptoms and require different treatment strategies. Limited knowledge was also reported regarding the recommendation of non–FDA approved medications (bupropion and α-2 agonists). Therefore, PCPs tend to refer to specialists (e.g., child and adolescent psychiatrists, developmental-behavioral pediatricians, pediatric neurologists) when the first-line medications for ADHD are not successful in treating the disorder [3]. PCPs reported lack of adequate education in other domains, such as how to identify children who are in need of psychoeducational evaluation, how to obtain these evaluations from the school [49], which community resources are available, and how to provide family education [3].

Second, data pointed out on a limited collaboration between PCPs and mental health providers, because of a poor delineation of generalist–specialist responsibilities and inadequate communication [50]. For example, although many pediatricians think that it is their responsibility to identify and refer mental health conditions, such as ADHD, they do not think that it is their responsibility to treat them [50]. Many communities do not have access to enough mental health providers for consultation with the PCP and for referrals [51, 52], thus PCPs often perceive their mental health colleagues as inaccessible [1]. Sometimes, the families themselves perceive societal stigmatization with mental health system and are reluctant to follow-up with further evaluation or treatment within the mental health system [1, 53]. As a result, many children's health care needs fall through the cracks, despite their interactions with both specialists and generalists [1, 54].

Similar problems characterize existing collaboration between PCPs and schools. Like physicians, school personnel find ADHD both challenging and time-consuming. Although teachers and school counselors may spend enormous amounts of time on managing ADHD-related issues, they may have little accurate knowledge about ADHD diagnosis and treatment. They may be adversarial toward PCPs who require services for their patients or do not provide clear communication of results [55].

Third, logistic factors, such as time pressures and lack of reimbursements, further complicate the implementation of AAP guidelines [44, 49, 56, 57]. Adequate evaluation of ADHD is time-consuming and requires the integration of information from multiple sources. It is estimated that initial evaluation for ADHD takes 2.5 - 8 hours [58], which sharply contrasts the typical 7-20 minute pediatric visits [49]. As a result, most PCPs do not have the necessary time to make an accurate diagnosis and discuss treatment options. A recent study including 21 urban and suburban practices [59], found that pediatric clinicians often presented information to persuade families to accept their preferred treatment instead of suggesting all options first. In contrast, families preferred comprehensive, unbiased information before decision making, even if they ultimately left the decision to the clinician [59, 60]. Another logistic problem commonly reported by PCPs is the lack of established, direct mechanisms for communication between the physician and other care providers, which make it difficult to collect information from a second source (such as the school) [61, 62]. A recurrent theme expressed by PCPs is the need for a team member or a "point person" (e.g., nurse, school worker, mental health specialist) to assist in collaborating with schools, educating families, and working with mental health care services [3]. Furthermore, limited financial resources, such as insurance constrain and lack of reimbursement [63], make it difficult to provide adequate care. For example, the California Medical Association reported that the majority (more than 70%) of primary care offices were operating at a fiscal deficit, given reimbursement rates under managed care [64]. It has been shown that urban PCPs experience substantially greater challenges with assessing ADHD and using FDA-approved medications than suburban PCPs, probably because they experience more problems in getting information from urban low-income schools and receiving consistent feedback from parents and teachers in monitoring medications [3, 33]. Also, urban PCPs who practice in clinics that are not affiliated with tertiary care hospitals may have fewer resources, which could make it more challenging for them to manage ADHD than other PCP who practice in hospital-affiliated programs [3].

In summary, AAP asserted that it is the pediatrician's responsibility to identify and treat ADHD. Significant efforts have been made to educate pediatricians about ADHD, including the distribution of a tool-kit designed specifically for primary care pediatrics [21]. Because ADHD has been addressed in a more organized and focused effort than any other behavioral and mental health problem commonly seen in pediatric settings, PCPs take more ownership of this mental health problem [42, 50]. However, there is still a substantial gap between the AAP recommendations and the capacity to provide ADHD services in the context of primary care practice.

Table 2. Potential Barriers to the Implementing of AAP Guidelines in Primary Care Practice

Category	Barriers
Lack of knowledge and training	Lack of formal training about the diagnosis and treatment of ADHD. Limited knowledge about recognizing coexisting mental health conditions. Limited knowledge about non–FDA approved medications. Limited information about how to identify children who are in need of psychoeducational evaluation. Limited knowledge how to obtain school evaluation. Limited knowledge about family education.
Limited collaboration with mental health providers	Poor delineation of generalist–specialist responsibilities and inadequate communications. Lack of access to enough mental health providers for consultation.
Logistic barriers	Lack of adequate time to make a diagnosis and discuss treatment options. Lack of established mechanisms for communication between physician and other care providers such as mental health specialists and school. Financial factors (e.g., insurance constraint, low-income communities, lack of reimbursement).

The AAP-recommended ADHD practice behaviors are quite complex to implement in a typical primary care setting. In order to implement the guidelines' recommendations, PCPs must have the background knowledge to use appropriate measurements for ADHD assessment and treatment monitoring. PCP must take time to educate parents about the need to collect parent and teacher ratings of their child's behavior, to collect ratings from parents and teachers and to score them. Finally, the PCP needs to interpret the rating scales in order to determine the presence of ADHD symptoms or the efficacy of treatment. In addition to being a complex process, this effort typically goes un- or under-reimbursed [65]. Thus, there is a consensus between researchers and clinicians that additional steps must be taken to allow implementation of the AAP guidelines in primary care settings [49, 66, 67]. In addition to provider education and the distribution of tools, focus should be given to improving collaboration between PCPs and other care providers to ensure the quality of care for children with ADHD in primary care settings.

IMPROVING THE ADHERENCE TO AAP GUIDELINES IN THE COMMUNITY PRACTICE

Implementing the AAP ADHD guidelines in a primary care practice is a complicated task that requires coordination of professionals on multiple levels. Many authors have warranted that implementation of evidence based practice into real-world service settings may fail unless factors such as PCPs' level of training in ADHD, comfort with managing mental health issues, and availability of mental health providers, are addressed in the long-term design of health care delivery [38, 43, 49, 68]. Since the publication of AAP guidelines, several efforts have been directed at assisting community-based providers to adhere to these guidelines. These programs focused on improving PCP's knowledge and comfort regarding the diagnosis and treatment of ADHD as well as improving collaboration between PCPs, mental health providers, families, and the education system.

One of the efforts assigned to improve AAP adherence was a quality improvement initiative called the ADHD Collaborative, which promotes the collaboration between community-based physicians (e.g., pediatricians) and mental health professionals (e.g., psychiatrists), in the Greater Cincinnati region [38]. Collaborative consultation service models use experts in mental health to score and interpret behavioral ratings collected by the pediatrician during assessment, titration of medication, or medication maintenance. Efficacy studies demonstrated that children treated by pediatricians who successfully adopted a consultation service showed large improvements in parent-and teacher-rated ADHD symptoms, than children treated by pediatricians who did not have access to these services. However; no group differences were found in functional impairment [38, 68]. Nevertheless, many pediatricians either failed to use the collaborative consultation services entirely or did not take full advantage of collaborative consultation services, especially regarding periodic treatment monitoring during medication maintenance. Authors concluded that because many children with ADHD continued to have significant functional impairment despite symptom improvement, collaboration with other mental health or educational services in addition to medication are warranted [38, 68].

One proposed solution to the unavailability of mental health professionals is to deliver mental health services in primary care settings [40, 69]. For instance, Kolko and co-workers [70] developed an integrative model collaborating mental health services for ADHD in primary care. The care model included an office-based nurse-administered intervention in primary care, which provided on-site psycho-education and cognitive behavioral therapy for children and families. Results from a randomized trial showed that the intervention program was advantaged over usual care (a referral to a local mental health provider) in reducing ADHD symptoms.

A plausible route to address the gap between primary care practice and AAP guidelines is the establishment of PCPs collaboration with the educational system. Foy et al. [55] described two case studies of community collaborative processes between elementary school personnel and community health care providers in the United States. The program is based on multiagency community group meetings (including education and health care of children as well as local parent support and advocacy groups) aimed to achieve consensus regarding assessment and treatment of children. As a result of this process, a shared consensus was achieved regarding ideal ADHD assessment, treatment, and management principles (facilitated by the AAP guidelines), including an agreed entry point at schools for children needing assessment, forms for collecting and exchanging information at every step, and key contacts (e.g., school nurse) for flow of communication at every step. Such collaboration is essential for addressing barriers to adequate care, such as pressures from parents and schools to prescribe stimulants and cultural biases that might affect the assessment of ADHD in school or families' help-seeking behavior. Collaboration between PCPs and school personnel may also improve the collection of data and school-physician communications, thereby decreasing physicians' non–face-to face (and thus non reimbursable) elements of care [55].

Bridging the Gap between Primary Care and Service Agencies: The Tertiary Care Model

ADHD is characterized by heterogeneity, ambiguity, and high comorbidity, and thus cannot lend itself to a universal treatment package. Because no single intervention is maximally effective, the literature supports a multimodal approach [20, 71-74]. An optimal multimodal model of care would have available comprehensive services, including mental health, education, social services, and the community from which the family and professional could select according to need. Inherent to the multimodal model is collaborative and integrated assessment, case planning, advocacy, management, and therapeutic services [75]. Putting all recommendations together, it is clear that innovative models are required to improve the diagnosis and treatment of children and adolescents with ADHD. One possible model involves shifting the focus from one in which individual psychiatrists provide direct services to children and families to one in which psychiatrists are engaged in consultative and collaborative care activities with pediatricians [51]. The specialization of mental health services for people with ADHD, provided by mental health services at a tertiary care level, offers a way forward.

Tertiary care is generally defined as specialized interventions delivered by highly trained professionals to individuals with problems that are particularly complex and difficult to treat in primary or secondary settings. It links community-based health care with multidisciplinary, regional, and tertiary pediatric care and is usually associated with academic activity.

Such a solution could be useful in overcoming the bureaucratic barriers at all service levels. It would encourage sharing resources and expertise, allow continuity of care during transition (from childhood to adulthood and from secondary to primary care) and improve recovery. It is also likely to reduce the social and economic burden on individuals and local populations that it aims to serve. In addition, tertiary care model would address the need expressed by PCP to have available ADHD expert to assist with medication issues, address issues of comorbidity, and treat appropriate referrals.

Hazelwood and co-workers [76] proposed a structure of a tertiary model for treating children with complex behavioral difficulties, including ADHD with or without comorbid diagnoses. This model was based on interviews with a multidisciplinary team in a tertiary center in Canada including social worker, psychiatrist, education consultant, and psychologists. In contrast to many existing systems, this model highlights the role of a case manager. Commonly, children can enter the intervention model by various referrals such as psychiatrist, education consultant or a family psychologist. Based upon the professional's area of expertise, assessment and treatment flowed from this particular reference point, which creates a large variance in service. However, the model proposed by Hazelwood et al. [76] begins with a single point of entry with a clinical case manager, skilled in addressing ADHD and knowledgeable in team strengths and expertise. The role of the case manager is to collect information from multiple resources and tests and to integrate these assessments. From this comprehensive collection of information, the case manager would formulate an individualized multimodal package and build a team around the perceived needs of the child and family. The selected team would provide in-depth assessments of identified areas of need and collaboratively design a treatment package. The model has built-in feedback loops to ensure that the process was not rigid and could address emerging needs.

Because ADHD is a chronic condition, optimal care for the disorder could be informed by the principles of chronic care models, such as the one developed by Wagner [77, 78]. The components of this mode are based on the unique characteristics of chronic conditions. It highlights the importance of a family-centered system of care that provides accessible healthcare services and information to families, decision making support across the entire continuum of care (including both the community and tertiary care levels), and a shared decision-making aids in order to help patients and families make value based informed choices. In particular, this model includes ongoing education and support to primary care providers on the care requirements of the child.

The feasibility and efficacy of tertiary care in managing ADHD relatively to PCPs have still to be uncovered. Yet, this model provides better systematic and consistent service, which is client-centered and need driven, based on an effective and efficient using of resources.

CONCLUSION

ADHD is a serious cognitive and behavior disorder of childhood, which has the potential for lifelong consequences. Children with ADHD are prone to delinquency, crime, substance abuse, and traffic accidents [79]. Among adults, impairment from ADHD can lead to additional missed work days, difficulty accomplishing tasks in the workplace, and less job stability [80]. However, such social, economic, and health costs could be preventable by an early and accurate diagnosis, a multi-pronged treatment approach, and continuing outcome research [81]. The AAP guidelines affirmed the critical role of primary care providers in the delivery of services to children with ADHD. Currently, PCPs take more ownership of ADHD than other mental health conditions [42, 50], but they encounter multiple barriers in providing adequate care for children and their families. These barriers include PCPs' limited knowledge and experience in managing ADHD, lack of time and financial resources to provide efficient care, poor communication with education professionals, and lack of availability of mental health professionals that could support primary care settings. Tertiary centers may provide a promising solution to these shortcomings, as they allow collaboration between all service systems and reduce the need of referrals to outside providers, such as local mental health clinics. There seems to be a benefit to using a case manager that would serve as a unique point of entree, collect comprehensive information, and receive constant feedback to allow the flexibility of the intervention plan. This kind of care model could ensure not only a parsimonious, shortened process of diagnosis and treatment but also a patient-centered intervention that would take into account individuals' needs and preferences.

REFERENCES

[1] Bunik M, Talmi A, Stafford B, Beaty B, Kempe A, Dhepyasuwan N, et al. Integrating mental health services in primary care continuity clinics: A national CORNET study. *Acad. Pediatr.* 2013;13:551–557.

[2] Hoagwood K, Kelleher KJ, Feil M, Comer DM. Treatment services for children with ADHD: a national perspective. *J Am Acad Child Adolesc Psychiatry.* 2000;39:198–206.

[3] Power TB, Mautone JA, Manz PH, Frye L, Nathan J. Managing Attention-Deficit/Hyperactivity Disorder in primary care: A systematic analysis of roles and challenges. *Pediatrics.* 2008;121:65-72.

[4] Swanson JM, Sergeant JA, Taylor E, Sonuga-Barke EJ, Jensen PS, Cantwell DP. Attention-deficit hyperactivity disorder and hyperkinetic disorder. *Lancet.* 1998; 351:429-433.

[5] Wolraich ML. Current assessment and treatment practices. In: Proceedings of the NIH consensus conference on diagnosis and treatment of ADHD. Bethesda, MD: *National Institutes of Health*; 1998. p.221–225.

[6] Biederman J. Mick E, Faraone SV. Age-dependent decline of symptoms of attention deficit hyperactivity disorder: impact of remission definition and symptom type. *Am. J. Psychiatry.* 2000;157: 816-818.

[7] Spencer TJ, Biederman J, Wilens TE, Faraone SV. Overview and Neurobiology of attention-deficit/hyperactivity disorder. *J. Clin. Psychiatry.* 2002; 63:3-9.

[8] Cole R, Mostofsky SH, Larson JCG, Denckla MB, Mahone EM. Age-related changes in motor subtle signs among girls and boys with ADHD. *Neurology.* 2008; 71: 1514–1520.

[9] Berger I, Nevo Y. Early developmental cues for diagnosis of attention deficit/hyperactivity disorder in young children. *Dev. Disabil. Res. Rev.* 2011; 17: 170-179.

[10] Kinsbourne M. Minimal brain dysfunction as a neurodevelopmental lag. *Ann. N. Y. Acad. Sci.* 1973; 205: 268-273.

[11] Shaw P, Eckstrand K, Sharp W, Blumenthal J, Lerch JP, Greenstein D et al. Attention-deficit/hyperactivity disorder is characterized by a delay in cortical maturation. *Proc. Natl. Acad. Sci.* 2007; 104:19649–19654.

[12] Shaw P, Malek M, Watson B, Sharp W, Evans A, Greenstein D. Development of cortical surface area and gyrification in attention-deficit/hyperactivity disorder. *Biol. Psychiatry.* 2012;72:191–197.

[13] Shevell M, Ashwal S, Donley D, Flint J, Gingold M, Hirtz D et al. Practice parameter: evaluation of the child with global developmental delay: report ofthe Quality Standards Subcommittee of the American Academy of Neurology and the Practice Committee of the Child Neurology Society. *Neurology.* 2003; 60:367–380.

[14]   Gustafsson P, Holmström E, Besjakov J, Karlsson MK. ADHD symptoms and maturity - a follow-up study in school children. *Acta Paediatr.* 2010; 99: 1536-1539.

[15]   Gjaerum B, Bjornerem H. Psychosocial impairment is significant in young referred children with and without psychiatric diagnoses and cognitive delays: applicability and reliability of diagnoses in face of co-morbidity. *Eur. Child Adolesc. Psy.* 2003;12:239-248.

[16]   Sonuga-Barke EJ, Halperin JM. Developmental phenotypes and causal pathways in attention deficit/hyperactivity disorder: potential targets for early intervention? *J. Child Psychol. Psychiatry.* 2010; 51:368–389.

[17]   Brown RT, Freeman WS, Perrin JM, Stein MT, Amler RW, Feldman HM, et al. Prevalence and assessment of attention-deficit/hyperactivity disorder in primary care settings. *Pediatrics.* 2001;107:e43.

[18]   Costello EJ, Costello AJ, Edelbrock C, Burns BJ, Dulcan MK, Brent D, Janiszewski S. Psychiatric disorders in pediatric primary care. *Arch. Gen. Psychiatry.* 1988;45:1107–1116.

[19]   Barkley RA. Attention-Deficit Hyperactivity Disorder: *A Handbook for Diagnosis and Treatment.* 2nd ed. New York: Guilford; 1998.

[20]   Jensen PS, Hinshaw SP, Swanson JM, Greenhill LL, Conners CK, Arnold LE, et al. Findings from the NIMH Multimodal Treatment Study of ADHD (MTA): implications and applications for primary care providers. *J. Dev. Behav. Pediatr.* 2001; 22:60-73.

[21]   American Academy of Pediatrics Subcommittee on Attention-Deficit/Hyperactivity Disorder and Committee on Quality and Improvement. Clinical practice guideline: treatment of the school-age child with attention-deficit/hyperactivity disorder. *Pediatrics.* 2001;108:1033–1044.

[22]   Burns BJ, Costello EJ, Angold A, Tweed D, Stangl D, Farmer EM, et al. Children's mental health service use across service sectors. *Health Aff* (Millwood). 1995;14:147-159.

[23]   Leaf PJ, Alegria M, Cohen P, Goodman SH, Horwitz SM, Hoven CW, et al. Mental health service use in the community and schools: results from the four-community MECA Study. Methods for the Epidemiology of Child and Adolescent Mental Disorders Study. *J. Am. Acad. Child Adolesc. Psychiatry.* 1996;35:889-897.

[24]   Mittal R, Sciberras E, Sewell J, Efron D. Assessment of children with learning and behavioural problems: Comparison of a multidisciplinary and sole paediatrician model. *J. Paediatr. Child Health.* 2013. doi:10.1111/jpc.12416

[25]   Cantwell DP. Attention deficit disorder: A review of the past 10 years. J. Am. Acad. Child Adolesc. *Psychiatry.* 1996; 35:978–987.

[26]   Kazdin AE. Psychosocial treatments for conduct disorder in children and adolescents. In: Nathan P, Gorman J, editors. A guide to treatments that work. 2nd ed. New York, NY: Oxford University Press; 2002. p.57–85.

[27]   Bureau of Health Professions. Shortage designation. 2004. Available from: http://bhpr.hrsa.gov/shortage.

[28]   Stevens S. Attention deficit/hyperactivity disorder: working the system for better diagnosis and treatment. *J. Pediatr. Nurs.* 2005;20:47-51.

[29]   Wasserman R, Kelleher KJ, Bocian A, Baker A, Childs GE, Indacochea F, et al. Identification of attentional and hyperactivity problems in primary care: a report from

Pediatric Research in Office Settings and the Ambulatory Sentinel Practice Network. *Pediatrics*. 1999;103: e38.

[30] Centers for Disease Control. (2004). CDC funds three research institutions to conduct population-based research on ADHD in children. Available from:www.cdc.gov/ncbddd/adhd/ institutes.htm.

[31] The Washington Post. Spending for children's behavioral medications rises.2004, May 17. Available from: Washingtonpost.com.

[32] Arnold L. Contemporary diagnosis and management of attention-deficit hyperactivity disorder. (2nd ed.). Newtown, PA: Handbooks in Health Care; 2002.

[33] Barkley R A. Psychosocial treatments for attention deficit/ hyperactivity disorder in children. *J. Clin. Psychiatry*. 2002; 63: 36– 43.

[34] Szymanski M, Zolotor A. Attention-deficit/hyperactivity disorder: Management. *Am. Fam. Physician*. 2001;64: 1355–1362.

[35] Scheffler RM, Brown TT, Fulton BD, Hinshaw SP, Levine P, Stone S. Positive association between attention-deficit/hyperactivity disorder medication use and academic achievement during elementary school. *Pediatrics*. 2009;123: 1273-1279.

[36] Hinshaw SP, Henker B, Whalen CK, Erhardt D, Dunnington RE Jr. Aggressive, prosocial, and nonsocial behavior in hyperactive boys: dose effects of methylphenidate in naturalistic settings. *J. Consult Clin. Psychol*. 1989;57:636-643.

[37] Abikoff H, Gittelman R. Hyperactive children treated with stimulants: is cognitive training a useful adjunct? *Arch. Gen. Psychiatry*. 1985;42:953-961.

[38] Epstein JN, Langberg JM, Lichtenstein PK, Altaye M, Brinkman WB, House K, et al. Attention-Deficit/Hyperactivity Disorder (ADHD) outcomes for children treated in community-based pediatric settings. *Arch. Pediatr. Adolesc. Med*. 2010; 164:160–165.

[39] Goldman LS, Genel M, Bezman RJ, Slanetz PJ. Diagnosis and treatment of attention-deficit/hyperactivity disorder in children and adolescents. Council on Scientific Affairs, American Medical Association. *JAMA*. 1998; 279:1100-1107.

[40] American Academy of Pediatrics. Clinical practice guideline: diagnosis and evaluation of the child with attention-deficit/hyperactivity disorder. *Pediatrics*. 2000; 105:1158–1170.

[41] Herrerias CT, Perrin JM, Stein MT. The child with ADHD: using the AAP clinical practice guideline. American Academy of Pediatrics. *Am. Fam. Physician*. 2001;63:1803–1810.

[42] Stein MT, Perrin JM. Diagnosis and treatment of ADHD in school-age children in primary care settings: a synopsis of the AAP practice guidelines. *Pediatr. Rev*. 2003; 24:92–98.

[43] Chan E, Hopkins MR, Perrin JM, Herrerias C, Homer CJ. Diagnostic practices for attention deficit hyperactivity disorder: A national survey of primary care physicians. *Ambulatory Pediatrics*. 2005;5:201–208.

[44] Rushton JL, Fant KE, Clark SL. Use of practice guidelines in the primary care of children with attention-deficit/hyperactivity disorder. *Pediatrics*. 2004;114: 23-28.

[45] Costello EJ, Angold A, Burns BJ, Stangl DK, Tweed DL, Erkanli A, Worthman CM. The Great Smoky Mountains Study of Youth: Goals, design, methods, and the prevalence of DSM III- R disorders. *Arch. Gen. Psychiatry*. 1996;53:1129–1136.

[46] Foley HA, Carlton CO, Howell RJ. The relationship of attention deficit hyperactivity disorder and conduct disorder to juvenile delinquency: legal implications. *Bull. Am. Acad. Psychiatry Law.* 1996; 24:333–345.

[47] Wolraich ML, Lambert EW, Bickman L, Simmons T, Doffing MA, Worley KA. Assessing the impact of parent and teacher agreement on diagnosing attention-deficit hyperactivity disorder. *J. Dev. Behav. Pediatr.* 2004;25:41–47.

[48] National Institutes of Health. Diagnosis and treatment of attention deficit/hyperactivity disorder (ADHD). *NIH Consens Statement.* 1998;16: 1–37.

[49] Leslie LK, Weckerly J, Plemmons D, Landsverk J, Eastman S. Implementing the American Academy of Pediatrics attention deficit/hyperactivity disorder diagnostic in primary care settings. *Pediatrics.* 2004;114:129–140.

[50] Heneghan A, Garner AS, Storfer-Isser A, Kortepeter K, Stein RE, Horwitz SM.. Pediatricians' role in providing mental health care for children and adolescents: do pediatricians and child adolescent psychiatrists agree? *J. Dev. Behav. Pediatr.* 2008;29:262–269.

[51] McCarthy M, Abenojar J, Anders TF. Child and adolescent psychiatry for the future: Challenges and opportunities. *Psychiatr. Clin. North Am.* 2009; 32: 213–226.

[52] Stiffman AR, Stelk W, Horwitz SM, Evans ME, Outlaw FH, Atkins M. A public health approach to children's mental health services: Possible solutions to current service inadequacies. *Adm. Policy Ment. Hlth.* 2010; 37:120-124.

[53] Pescosolido BA, Perry BL, Martin JK, McLeod JD, Jensen PS. Stigmatizing attitudes and beliefs about treatment and psychiatric medications for children with mental illness. *Psychiatr. Serv.* 2007;58:613–618.

[54] Finkelstein JA, Lozano P, Shulruff R, Inui TS, Soumerai SB, Ng M, et al. Self-reported physician practices for children with asthma: are national guidelines followed? *Pediatrics.* 2000;106 :886–896.

[55] Foy JM, Earls MF. A process for developing community consensus regarding the diagnosis and management of attention-deficit/hyperactivity disorder. *Pediatrics.* 2005;115: 97-104.

[56] Simonian SJ. Screening and identification in pediatric primarycare. *Behav. Modif.* 2006;30:114–131.

[57] Weitzman CC, Leventhal JM. Screening for behavioral health problems in primary care. *Curr. Opin. Pediatr.* 2006;18: 641–648.

[58] Robin AL. ADHD in adolescents: Diagnosis and treatment. New York: The Guilford Press; 1998.

[59] Fiks A, Hughes CC, Gafen A, Guevara, JP, Barg FK. Contrasting Parents' and Pediatricians' Perspectives on Shared Decision-Making in ADHD. *Pediatrics.* 2011; 127: 188–196.

[60] Jackson D, Peters K. Use of drug therapy in children with attention deficit hyperactivity disorder (ADHD): maternal views and experiences. *J. Clin. Nurs.* 2008; 17, 2725-2732.

[61] Jerome L, Gordon M, Hustler P. A comparison of American and Canadian teachers' knowledge and attitudes towards attention deficit hyperactivity disorder (ADHD). *Can. J. Psychiatry.* 1994;39:563–567.

[62] Wolraich ML, Lindgren S, Stromquist A, Milich R, Davis C, Watson D. Stimulant medication use by primary care physicians in the treatment of attention deficit hyperactivity disorder. *Pediatrics.* 1990;86:95–101.

[63] Leslie LK, Stallone K, Weckerly J, McDaniel AL, Monn A. Implementing the ADHD guidelines in primary care: does one size fit all? *J. Health Care Poor Underserve.* 2006;17:302–327.

[64] California medical association. The coming medical group failure epidemic: Access to m Care for millions of Californians is at risk. San Francisco, CA: California Medical Association; 1999.

[65] Epstein JN, Langberg JM, Lichtenstein PK, Kolb R, Altaye M, Simon JO. Use of an Internet portal to improve community-based pediatric ADHD care: a cluster randomized trial. *Pediatrics.* 2011; 28: 1201-208.

[66] National advisory mental health council workgroup on child and adolescent mental health intervention development and deployment. Blueprint for change: research on child and adolescent mental health. Washington, DC: *National Institute of Mental Health*; 2001

[67] Hoagwood K, Burns BJ, Kiser L, Ringeisen H, Schoenwald SK. Evidence-based practice in child and adolescent mental health services. *Psychiatr. Serv.* 2001;52:1179–1189.

[68] Epstein JN, Rabiner D, Johnson DE, Fitzgerald DP, Chrisman A, Erkanli A, et al.. Improving Attention-Deficit/Hyperactivity Disorder treatment outcome through use of a collaborative consultation treatment service by community based pediatricians: A cluster randomized trial. *Arch. Pediatr. Adolesc. Med.* 2007; 161:835–840.

[69] Kelleher K, Campo J, Gardner W. Management of pediatric mental disorders in primary care: where are we now and where are we going? *Curr. Opin. Pediatrics.* 2006;18:649–653.

[70] Kolko DJ, Campo JV, Kilbourne AM, Kelleher K. Doctor-office collaborative care for pediatric behavioral problems: a preliminary clinical trial. *Arch. Pediatr. Adolesc. Med.* 2012;166:224-231.

[71] Arnold LE, Abikoff HB, Cantwell DP, Conners CK, Elliott G, Greenhill LL, et al. National Institute of Mental Health collaborative multimodal treatment study of children with ADHD (the MTA).*Arch Gen Psychiatry.* 1997; 54: 865–870.

[72] Ialongo N, Horn W, Pascoe J, Greenberg G, Packard T, Lopez M, et al.The effects of a multimodal intervention with attention-deficit hyperactivity disorder children: a 9 month follow-up. *J. Am. Academy Child Adolesc. Psychiatr.* 1993; 38: 182–189.

[73] Richters JE, Arnold LE, Jensen PS, Abikoff H, Conners CK, Greenhill LL, et al. NIMH collaborative multisite multimodal treatment study of children with ADHD: I. Background and rationale. *J. Am. Acad. Child Adolesc. Psychiatry.* 1995; 34:987-1000.

[74] Pelham W, Wheeler, Chronis A. Empirically supported psychosocial treatments for attention deficit hyperactivity disorder. *J. Clin. Child Psychol.* 1998; 27:190–205.

[75] Taylor M. Attention-deficit hyperactivity disorder on the frontlines: management in the primary care office. *Compr. Ther.* 1999; 25: 313–325.

[76] Hazelwood E, Bovingdon T, Tiemens K. The meaning of a multimodal approach for children with ADHD: experiences of service professionals. *Child Care Health Dev.* 2002 ;28:301-307.

[77] Wagner EH, Austin BT, Davis C, Hindmarsh M, Schaefer J, Bonomi A. Improving chronic illnesscare: translating evidence into action. *Health Aff* (Millwood). 2001;20:64–78.

[78] Bodenheimer T, Wagner EH, Grumbach K. Improving primary care for patients with chronic illness. *JAMA*. 2002; 288 :1775–1779.

[79] Matza LS, Paramore C, Prasad M.A review of the economic burden of ADHD. *Cost Eff Resour Alloc*. 2005; 3: 5.

[80] Birnbaum HG, Kessler RC, Lowe SW, Secnik K, Greenberg PE, Leong SA, Swensen AR.

[81] Costs of attention deficit-hyperactivity disorder (ADHD) in the US: excess costs of persons with ADHD and their family members in 2000. *Curr. Med. Res. Opin*. 2005;21:195-206.

[82] Wilens TE, Faraone SV, Biederman J, Gunawardene S. Does stimulant therapy of attention-deficit/hyperactivity disorder beget later substance abuse? A meta-analytic review of the literature. *Pediatrics*. 2003; 111:179–185.

In: ADHD
Editors: Itai Berger and Adina Maeir

ISBN: 978-1-63321-047-9
© 2014 Nova Science Publishers, Inc.

Chapter 2

THE TEEN COG-FUN MODEL OF INTERVENTION FOR ADOLESCENTS WITH ADHD

Nirit Levanon-Erez and Adina Maeir, Ph.D.*
School of Occupational Therapy, Hadassah and Hebrew University

ABSTRACT

This chapter will present the application of the Cog-Fun intervention model (see chapter 6 in this book) to adolescents with ADHD. The chapter will include: (a) a discussion of the unique issues of adolescents with ADHD; (b) hypothesized enabling factors that promote satisfying participation in life roles and quality of life, factors that will be presented from Occupational Therapy (OT) and cognitive rehabilitation conceptual models that provide a theoretical framework for understanding and addressing the challenges of adolescents with ADHD; and (c) the proposed integrative Teen Cog-Fun treatment protocol along with case studies to illustrate the treatment process and enabling factors.

INTRODUCTION: ADHD AND ADOLESCENCE

Attention deficit hyperactivity disorder (ADHD) contains two main types of symptoms: inattention and hyperactive-impulsive behavior (APA, 2000). According to Barkley (2006) and Brown (2013), ADHD is in essence a neurocognitive disorder seen as a developmental impairment of executive functions (EFs) which are defined as self - regulatory processes responsible for the individual's goal directed behavior (Barkley, 2012). There is strong evidence supporting the presence of executive dysfunction in ADHD (Willcut, Doyle, Nigg, Faraone, & Pennington, 2005), which puts individuals at high risk for significant long-term limitations and negative outcomes in broad areas of occupational functioning (Biederman, et al., 2004; Brown, 2009). ADHD was initially considered a developmental disorder of

---

* Correspondence: Nirit Levanon-Erez MSc OT School of Occupational Therapy, Hadassah and Hebrew University PO Box 24026, Mount Scopus, Jerusalem, 91240, E-mail: niriterez1@gmail.com.

childhood that gradually resolves during adolescence. However, this view has been contradicted by systematic follow-up studies documenting the persistence of ADHD across the lifespan (Biederman, Petty, Evans, Small, & Faraone, 2010; Geissler, & Lesch, 2011). The understanding of ADHD as a chronic disorder has led to a life transition model which defines crucial transition points in adolescence and young adulthood that require special attention and care (Turgay, et al., 2012).

Adolescence is a critical stage of development. Adolescents seek autonomy and independence and are expected to take more responsibility in managing their occupations. Concurrently, complexity and load in all occupational roles increases. The academic requirements in school grow both quantitatively and qualitatively. The participation in organized leisure activities becomes more specialized, demanding higher levels of performance and commitment (e.g., sports, arts, youth organizations). Participation in instrumental activities of daily living (IADL) is expanded to include activities such as money management, health management and driving. The developmental process of their significant social relationships involves a shift from parental dependency to more equal relationships with parents and a growing emphasis on peer relationships (De Goede , Branje, & Meeus, 2009; Rubin, Bukowski, & Parker, 2006). Social participation with peers requires a high level of social skills to understand the ever-changing social cues and codes and respond to them appropriately. In summary, adolescence is characterized by increasing demands in many occupational areas which may be even more challenging for an adolescent with ADHD due to an increasing imbalance between demands and resources (Turgay, et al., 2012). The neurocognitive profile of ADHD comprising attention and executive deficits, are especially vulnerable to task complexity, load and novelty (Brown, 2006). Task demands in occupational roles are greater than their abilities; hence participation is not congruent with their expectations and those of their social frameworks. Therefore, adolescents experience increasing challenges and recurrent failures and frustration. There is growing evidence documenting these difficulties of adolescents with ADHD in multiple domains. Academically, adolescents with ADHD demonstrate lower levels of achievement, higher rates of grade retention and increased risk for school dropout (Barbaresi, Katusic, Colligan, Weaver, & Jacobsen, 2007; Barkley, Fischer, Smallish, & Fletcher, 2006; Frazier, Youngstrom, Glutting, & Watkins, 2007). The social participation of adolescents with ADHD is characterized by more aggressive and antisocial behaviors, poor social skills, impaired abilities to accurately gauge their social and behavioral competence, social-cognitive deficits (social comprehension, social problem-solving) and elevated peer rejection (Murray-Close et al., 2010; Sibley, Evans, & Serpell, 2010). Within the family context, adolescents with ADHD and their parents experience more conflict, more anger in these conflicts, more aggressive conflict tactics, and poorer communication than typical adolescents. Parents of adolescents with ADHD have been shown to perceive their child's behaviors in negative ways and themselves as lacking power. Adolescents have been shown to experience parent rejection and hostility (Edwards, Barkley, Laneri, Fletcher, & Metevia, 2001; Glatz, Stattin, & Kerr, 2011; Lifford, Harold, & Thapar, 2008; 2009). The strained parent-adolescent relationship impedes the adequate fulfillment of the parenting role which further hinders adolescent development.

In light of all the difficulties presented above, the adolescent's psychological well-being is compromised with diminished sense of competency and self-efficacy. Furthermore, ADHD is associated with increased risk for a wide range of psychiatric disorders including, mood disorders, anxiety disorders, eating disorders and personality disorders (Yoshimasu et al., 2012). Youth with ADHD are also at risk to become involved in deviant activities, including substance use (Elkins, McGue, & Iacono, 2007; Gudjonsson, Sigurdsson, Sigfusdottir, & Young, 2012; Wilens, et al., 2011), early initiation of sexual behavior (Flory, Molina, Pelham, Gnagy, & Smith, 2006), risky driving (Barkley & Cox, 2007) and delinquency (Sibley, et al., 2011).

Successful adaptation to ADHD is compromised by youth's insufficient knowledge and awareness of their ADHD. In the neurocognitive rehabilitation literature, self-awareness refers to one's knowledge and recognition of the neurological health condition, its symptoms and consequential functional disabilities (Katz, & Maeir, 2011; Kortte, & Wegener, 2004; Toglia, & Kirk, 2000). Adolescents have been found to underestimate the severity of their ADHD symptoms relative to parent and teacher reports, to cognitive measures of impulsiveness and inattention and to professional medical diagnosis of ADHD (Danckaerts, Heptinstall, Chadwick, & Taylor, 1999, Sibley et al., 2012; Smith, Pelham, Gnagy, Molina, & Evans, 2000; Young, et al., 2010). Furthermore, adolescents were shown to underrate their level of functional impairment (Sibley et al., 2012), their social problems (Murray-Close et al., 2010) and their everyday performance, especially in applied cognition domains, such as "dealing with difficult situations" and "remembering homework (Volz-Sidiropoulou, Boecker, & Gauggel, 2013). This lack of awareness in the face of repeated negative feedback may generate confusion, reduced sense of coherence and control and adversely affect positive adjustment to ADHD. In sum, this review demonstrates the broad impact of ADHD in adolescence, involving neurological and psychosocial barriers to participation in multiple occupational domains. Intervention programs are needed in order to help adolescents with ADHD cope with their challenges, minimize risks and promote their options for an adaptive, productive life as adults.

HYPOTHESIZED ENABLING FACTORS

The life transition model for ADHD emphasizes that the key to successful functioning can be conceptualized as a balance between environmental demands and available resources (Turgay, et al., 2012). The focus of treatment programs should be on bridging this gap and restoring balance by a collaborative process in which the adolescent takes responsibility and feels ownership. Nevertheless, providing intervention for adolescents is challenging. Adolescents' deficient awareness of ADHD and deficient decision making processes as well as vulnerable self-esteem and need for autonomy, may compromise client collaboration in treatment. Accordingly, the reported adherence to ADHD treatment of adolescents is low (Bussing et al., 2012). Therefore, effective intervention programs must relate to the adolescent's individual perspective and tailor the treatment process to the client's unique profile.

According to the International Classification of Functioning Disability and Health (ICF) model of health implications (WHO, 2001), as well as the OT paradigm (Roley, et al., 2008), the primary health outcomes are satisfying engagement and participation in life roles and occupations whereby the person has an experience of congruency between demands and performance. The gold standard for intervention for ADHD involves the combination of pharmacological and psychosocial treatments (NIMH, 2008; NICE, 2008). The Teen Cog-Fun is a psychosocial, integrative OT practice model that is designed to enable the individual to cope effectively with ADHD in their occupational contexts. This model utilizes established OT models that explain the person and environment factors that contribute to occupational performance and guide intervention for individuals with chronic health conditions.

The teen Cog-Fun is based on the assumption that the central psychosocial enabling factors that promote positive coping with ADHD across the lifespan comprise: (a) *adaptive self-awareness* that is defined as the awareness of strengths and values in daily life, the recognition of ADHD symptoms and their implications in various occupations together with a sense of self efficacy. *Adaptive self-awareness* promotes occupational performance in several ways. Connecting to ones values and abilities fosters meaning and satisfaction, accurate knowledge and attribution of challenges enables the recruitment of appropriate resources. Together, these contribute to a sense of coherence, control and self-efficacy that motivate and guide appropriate goal setting and effective management of ADHD. Furthermore, *adaptive self-awareness* is especially important during the identity formation that occurs during adolescence; (b) *efficient cognitive strategy use* which refers to an organized cognitive approach, methods, or tactics that operate to compensate for executive deficits and guide efficient adaptive behavior. For example, a 'Plan Strategy' which includes systematic attention to task steps, and consequences compensates for impulsivity and poor planning; (c) *enabling environments* refers to the support and adaptations provided by the social environments of adolescents with ADHD. For example, parents' compassionate understanding and acceptance of challenges, appreciation of strengths and setting realistic expectations enable the adolescent to succeed and develop adaptive self-awareness. The teen Cog-Fun is designed to support the development of these three enabling factors, and by them to promote satisfying participation in life roles and quality of life for the adolescents and their families. Following is a brief discussion of the three OT and cognitive rehabilitation conceptual models that provide the foundation for the treatment principles and methods.

Model of Human Occupation (MOHO) (Kielhofner, 2008)

The MOHO model provides the overarching framework for the Teen Cog-Fun. This model provides a theoretical understanding of the factors that enable occupational performance and explains how occupation is motivated, patterned and performed. The MOHO broadly integrates human and environmental factors that shape occupational performance. In this model, humans are conceptualized as being made up of three interrelated components: (a) Volition, defined as the motivational foundation for occupation that originates in self-perception and awareness, values and interests; (b) Habituation, defined as the process by which occupation is organized into patterns or routines; (c) Performance capacity comprising the physical and mental abilities that underlie occupational performance. In he MOHO the physical and social environment in which occupation takes place are considered as important factors that can enable or restrict participation.

The Teen Cog-Fun model relies on the MOHO in several ways: first, the conceptualization of volition as the motivational foundation for occupation underlies the Teen Cog-Fun's objective to link occupational performance to volitional constructs. The definition of *adaptive self-awareness* is based on the conceptualization of volition, hence promoting *adaptive self-awareness* within the Teen Cog-Fun means promoting clients' knowledge of what they want in connection with their values, interests, desires and realistic understanding of strengths and weaknesses.

Furthermore, understanding and connecting to volitional constructs is especially relevant for the Teen Cog-Fun model since adolescents are preoccupied with developing their independent identity. In order for the intervention to be effective at this unique phase it must uncover and foster the adolescent's volitional entities and harness them to the change process. Finally, the understanding of the MOHO that environmental factors impact participation guides the assumption of the Teen Cog-Fun model that *enabling environments* is an essential part of intervention.

Bio–Psycho–Social (BPS) Theory of Awareness in Neurorehabilitation (Ownsworth, Clare, & Morris, 2006)

This theory explains the barriers to awareness in neurocognitive health conditions and provides a comprehensive account of the underlying mechanisms of unawareness in neuro-rehabilitation. The BPS theory emphasizes the interplay between neurological damage relating directly to the disease or injury and the psychological resources that the client brings to the situation, within a wider social context. The model is based on research conducted in non-ADHD neurological populations and provides an integrative and valuable theoretical foundation to examine the factors that may influence awareness in ADHD. The biological factor, directly stemming from the neurological involvement, causes neurocognitive deficits that preclude learning from experience. For example, an attention deficit prevents the person from perceiving feedback from performance, and executive deficit prevents reflecting and processing this feedback.

The psychological factor is attributed to defensive mechanisms created to protect the individual from psychic distress. These psychodynamic mechanisms prevent the painful emotional experiences associated with acknowledgement of difficulties. The social factor addresses the contextual views and beliefs towards a health condition, in the society as a whole as well as those held by the client's significant others, and the degree to which the diagnosis is openly discussed (Ownsworth et al., 2006). In the Teen Cog Fun, the understanding of these factors guides the treatment methods that target the development of *adaptive self-awareness*. These methods include manipulating these bio-psycho-social factors underlying awareness.

The biological neurocognitive factor that impedes awareness is addressed by guided monitoring and discovery of strengths and weaknesses in occupational performance. The therapeutic mediation during task performance bypasses the attention deficits and impulsivity which typically preclude awareness in the client's ongoing experiences.

The psychological factor is addressed by enabling success in occupational performance, highlighting strengths and gradual exposure to challenges which are linked to the discovery of strategies. Taken together this experience reduces the threat of recognizing difficulties and promotes acceptance and effective coping. The social factor is addressed by accessing information to the teen and parents, and guiding the parents to be a source of awareness for their child.

Multicontext Treatment Approach (MTA) (Toglia, 2011)

The MTA targets the development of strategies and self-awareness. This treatment approach was developed for neurocognitive rehabilitation populations and can be applicable to ADHD as ADHD is a neurocognitive disorder. The MTA is based on the Dynamic Interactional Model of Cognition (DIM) (Toglia, 2011). In the DIM, strategies are conceptualized as organized approaches, methods, or tactics that operate to compensate for neurocognitive deficits. For example highlighting key attributes of the task may compensate for poor attention to details, rehearsing details may compensate for poor working memory. Self-awareness supports the generation and use of strategies and includes two distinct but interrelated concepts: (a) self-knowledge which comprises the understanding of one's cognitive strengths and limitations, for example knowledge of cognitive deficits resulting from ADHD; (b) on-line awareness which refers to metacognitive skills that are activated during task performance, such as judging task demands, anticipating problems, monitoring, regulating and evaluating performance. In the DIM strategies and self-awareness are considered modifiable, thus are target for MTA intervention. Key elements of the MTA include strategy self-generation and explicit transfer training; enhancing self-monitoring and self-awareness; use of everyday activities that are tailored to the client's level and interests. These elements are hypothesized to enhance the probability of transfer of learning. In addition, the activity and environment can be modified to complement the individual change process, in order to optimize occupational performance. In the Teen Cog-Fun, the MTA guides the treatment methods for the development of cognitive strategies in occupational context.

The Teen Cog-Fun Protocol

The teen cog-fun protocol is designed to support the development of *adaptive self-awareness, cognitive strategies and enabling environments* in order to promote satisfying participation in life roles and quality of life for adolescents and their families. The intervention protocol includes four units (See Table A). Unit A is devoted entirely to the development of *adaptive self-awareness*. Initially the client is guided to study personal strengths through analysis of individual occupational profile and experience with cognitive tasks and games. Values are then discussed, based on the Portrait Values Questionnaire (PVQ) (Schwartz, Melech, Lehmann, Burgess, & Harris, 2001). This questionnaire is derived from the Basic Human Values theory (Schwartz, 1992), and measures the values of the respondent. The PVQ includes short verbal portraits of 40 different people, gender-matched with the respondent. Each portrait describes a person's goals, aspirations, or wishes that point implicitly to the importance of a value. For each portrait, respondents answer: "How much like you is this person? We infer respondents' own values from their self-reported similarity to people described implicitly in terms of particular values (Schwartz et al., 2001). The PVQ is analyzed with the client and their values are examined in relation to their everyday occupational experience. After the client discovers strengths and values, psycho- education regarding ADHD and EF is enabled through supported learning activities. Then, the client experiences ADHD implications during challenging therapeutic activities and simulations of real life occupations.

Table A. Summary of Intervention units

Unit	Aim	Objectives	Treatment methods
A	Develop adaptive self-awareness	(a) Discover strengths in occupational contexts (b) Link volition to occupational experience (c) Understand personal challenges resulting from ADHD and their impact on occupational performance	Analysis of individual occupational profile Simulation of daily occupations Experiences with cognitive tasks and games Analysis of the PVQ (Schwartz, et al. 2001) Guided learning of informational resources
B	Strategy acquisition in a functional context	(a) Acquire global strategies of Self-monitoring, Goal setting, Task analysis, Plan and Review. (b) Acquire specific executive strategies tailored to clients executive profile (e.g., list making, visual stop cue, breathing techniques, self-generated motivators)	Guided discovery and learning of strategies Practice of strategies within multiple contexts: cognitive activities and simulation of daily occupations Monitoring transfer of strategies to client-centered occupational goals
C.	Recruitment and adaptation of environmental resources	(a) Parents will promote adaptive self-awareness by providing specific positive feedback and attributing child's dysexecutive behaviors to ADHD (b) Parents will support teens self-management through collaborative goal setting (c) Parents will adapt expectations and implement supports for occupational performance	Parent –therapist collaborative learning sessions
D.	Promote transfer and generalization of treatment gains	(a) Consolidate the intervention process (b) Promote parent-teen collaboration in the implementation of strategies in everyday life	Preparing a creative project that summarizes personal profile, goals obtained and strategies acquired. Presenting and discussing the final project with the parents

Through this process the client formulates his personal profile that includes his challenges stemming from ADHD along with his strengths and values. At the end of the first unit the client is ready to formulate initial occupational goals that link the client's everyday occupations with his personal profile. In unit B, *cognitive strategies* are acquired in the context of these self-set goals. We distinguish between general and specific executive strategies. General strategies include (a) Self-monitoring strategy which supports the monitoring of performance during tasks as well as the monitoring of the task demands; (b)

Goal setting strategy– which supports the skill of defining specific, measurable and attainable goals; (c) Task analysis strategy – that includes identification of the action sequence, the necessary skills and relevant materials for performing a task; (d) Plan and review strategy – which is a general template for planning the execution of goal intentions and monitoring achievements. Specific strategies target various executive deficits, for example a visual stop reminder can target inhibition, self-generated motivators can target effort recruitment and list making can compensate for poor working memory. The client discovers these specific strategies through a mediated learning experience during activities that simulate his occupational goals. In Unit C, *enabling environments* is fostered by collaborative learning sessions with the parents. In these sessions the therapist provides knowledge and skills as needed for the parents to support their teen's adaptive awareness and self- management. The therapist guides the parents to provide specific positive feedback to their child and to attribute their child's dysexecutive behaviors to ADHD. In addition, the parents are encouraged to adjust their expectations, are trained in collaborative goal setting and in providing the necessary supports for successful occupational performance. Unit D summarizes the entire process and focuses on integrating the previous units. In this unit the adolescent prepares a creative project that summarizes his personal profile, goals obtained and strategies acquired. In the concluding session, the adolescent presents his final project to his parents, and then they discuss together how they can continue to implement the acquired tools to promote transfer and generalization. This session affords the opportunity to practice self-advocacy as well as to further recruit parental support. See Table A for a summary of the intervention units.

Case Studies

Case Study 1: Sara

Sara is 14. 6 years old, diagnosed with ADHD in elementary school for which she regularly takes medication. She is the oldest of five children in an orthodox family and currently attends a seminar for girls. According to Sara's parents her time management is very problematic and causes a lot of strain in the family. She is chronically late for seminar, extracurricular activities, appointments and chores. In addition they describe difficulties in social activities with family and friends, such as fighting with her younger brothers and difficulty maintaining friendships. Sara struggles with academic tasks at seminar and home, and requires private tutoring. Sara demonstrates marked strengths in arts, which she pursues in extracurricular activities and designing in the home. She also demonstrates good communication skills with cousins and parents when she is relaxed. The Behavior Rating Inventory of Executive Function (BRIEF) (Gioia, Isquith, Guy & Kenworthy, 2000) parent profile, indicated deficits in inhibition, emotional control, initiation, working memory and planning/organization (see table B1). Sara's parents identified occupational goals in the Canadian Occupational Performance Measures (COPM) (Law et al. , 2002), which were 'being on time', 'meeting friends more often', 'get along with siblings', 'doing homework and study for tests' (see table B2). The awareness interview with Sara revealed minimal awareness of ADHD symptoms and vague knowledge of strategies: "I don't really know what ADHD is. Sometimes I can't really concentrate. I don't want to be late. I want to get to places on time, in the morning, or to after school activities. I write down (what I want to do) but it doesn't work and I get stuck". Sara portrayed occupational identity dissatisfaction: "I'm not a hard worker. I don't know what I want to do when I grow up, maybe a designer. I hope it works out but you never know".

In the intervention process Sara's awareness to her strengths was targeted first. Sara's good visual memory and her talent for designing were discovered through cognitive games. Sara's skills in communication and arts were discovered through occupational analysis, Sara's gift for creating a pleasant atmosphere, her sensitivity to other people and sense of humor were discovered through analysis of her interactions in the therapeutic context. Next, based on analyzing the manifestations of the PVQ in daily life, Sara acknowledged the things that were important for her: to succeed in school, to care for family and friends, to engage in fun activities, like painting and spending time with friends and to be independent. Initially, Sara recognized the incongruence of her values with her daily activities. Gradually, during the therapeutic process, she was more able to integrate her values with her occupational performance. For example, her desire to succeed in school was integrated in her goals and she was able to access this value when managing her time (see below).

Following, psycho- education regarding ADHD was introduced; Sara watched videos and presentation containing explanations and personal stories, and was asked which symptoms resemble hers. Sara acknowledged her challenges: shift – "sometimes it's hard for me to change what I do", initiation– "I don't like to get up in the morning" "I do my schoolwork in the last minute" planning – "I usually don't decide when I should start getting ready". This discovery led to Sara's formulation of her goal: 'to improve my time management'. Following, she was guided to define more specific and attainable goals: Get to painting class on time; Get to seminar on time; be prepared for test on time (see table B3).

In working to achieve these goals Sara was taught the general task analysis strategy of analyzing task demands and personal requirements. In this process Sara's understanding of her challenges deepened: "I don't want to stop a fun activity in order to start one that I need to do"; "I don't like starting boring or difficult tasks". Based on this awareness Sara was able to generate new strategies and wrote her plan: "To get to painting class on time, I should decide that it's important, and then decide when I need to start getting ready". A week later, Sara reviewed her plan and realized that it didn't work because she didn't notice that the time to get ready had passed. Sara was guided to look for a strategy or adaptation and decided to ask her mother for a reminder. The next week Sara said that her mother agreed to help, but this plan worked only once, the second time she indeed did get ready on time but "once I was ready (to go out) I started doing something else and felt that I had plenty of time, and I ended up being late". Sara realized that she wasn't able to make accurate time estimations. In the next sessions Sara practiced estimating how long it would take her to perform different tasks. She generated a strategy of analyzing task's steps, and visualizing herself performing them. Sara used this strategy to figure out how long it would take her to get ready to go out. She estimated 20 minutes and decided to try and time herself. Sara wrote a new plan, "To get to painting class on time, I should decide that it's important, write down all the things I should do before I leave, ask for a reminder from my mother 20 minutes before I should leave, and time myself". This time Sara's plan was successful. Then Sara defined the strategies that she can use to achieve another goal: "I need to decide that the goal is important to me, plan for it in advance, and ask for help" Sara decided to use these strategies on her "be prepared for my test on time" goal. She wrote her plan " Decide that it's important, find out the test material, get it, go over test material and divide it to parts, estimate how long it would take me to study each part and make a time table, study with a friend". As mentioned above Sara began to experience greater integration of her values with her daily actions and goals.

To foster social support, the initial stage of parent guidance focused on connecting with Sara's strengths. Her parents began to realize that their perception of her was greatly influenced by the daily struggles of time management. They were very open to attending to her strengths and providing her with specific positive feedback. For example, they encouraged her expression of artistic design in her room and other designated areas in the house. Further on the parents learned to understand, that her executive challenges are related to her ADHD and were able to set more realistic goals for her. For example, the parents shifted their initial expectations that Sara 'always be on time' to 'being on time to seminar'. They also discovered effective supports for her time management (e.g., hanging up a clock, supplying reminders upon Sara's request).

The summary unit was an opportunity for Sara to consolidate her new learning. She prepared a poster presentation of her process in therapy. Her presentation demonstrated improved self-awareness, along with more confidence that she could set and achieve occupational goals that were significant to her. Her parents appeared to appreciate the steps she was taking along with her hard work. The family discussed the next steps to transfer these gains to their day-to-day life. Following intervention Sara and her parents reported clinically significant improvement (> 2 points on the COPM) in targeted goals, except for 'get along with siblings' (which was not a goal that Sara defined) (see tables B2 & B3). The parents ratings on the BRIEF also indicated a clinically significant improvement, with post-treatment scores below the impaired cutoff score (65) (See table B1).

Table B1. BRIEF parent profile

Executive Function	T score pre*	T score post*
Inhibit	70	55
Shift	56	45
Emotional control	70	61
Initiate	77	53
Working memory	77	58
Plan/organize	76	63
Organization of materials	53	47
Monitor	64	43
Behavior Regulation Index	69	55
Meta cognitive Index	75	55
Global Executive	73	55

* (>65 considered deficient).

Table B2. Parent's COPM

Goal	Performance Pre (1-10)	Performance Post* (1-10)
Being on time for seminar	3	6
Meeting friends more often	3	10
Get along with siblings	3	3
Doing homework	5	7
Study for tests	3	8

* (2 point change considered clinically significant).

Table B3. Sara's COPM

Goal	Performance Pre (1-10)	Performance Post (1-10)
Get to painting class on time	6. 5	9
Get to seminar on time	5	9
Be prepared for test on time.	5	8

Case Study 2: Ron

Ron is 15. 5 years old, and was diagnosed with ADHD in preschool. He is the youngest child in the family and is currently in the tenth grade. Ron doesn't take medication to control his ADHD due to a medical intolerance. Ron's Parents describe him as smart. They say he understands things easily and quickly. He is usually a happy child and has many friends. Ron is a talented basketball player who plays in the school and sports club teams. He spends a few hours every day in training. At school, Ron has behavioral issues; he interrupts in class, talks disrespectfully to teachers and often misses classes. Furthermore, Ron often doesn't do his homework and rarely studies for tests. He got caught copying a few times in tests and even got suspended once this year. When his parents offer to help him in schoolwork, Ron refuses to cooperate. At home, Ron spends a lot of time playing video games and has minimal communication and involvement with family members. He often refuses to perform domestic tasks and has many arguments with his parents. The parent BRIEF profile indicated deficits in inhibition, shift, emotional control, working memory planning/organization, organization of materials and monitoring. (See table C1). Ron's parents identified occupational goals in the COPM which were: 'to accept help in schoolwork', 'study for tests', 'perform domestic tasks', 'more involvement with family'. (See table C2).

The awareness interview with Ron revealed partial awareness of ADHD symptoms and strategies: "I'm very active all the time (hyperactive) but I say that I don't have ADHD and I can control 'it'. However, when people look at me and say: 'do you see yourself?' Then I get it. My teachers tell me that I move all the time and talk a lot, so I guess I have a problem. It's hard for me to sit and study for a long time. I don't have the energy for homework, I can do it but I don't think that it's important. I'm smart, I can succeed in school but I don't study for tests. I don't work hard. Sometimes my mom makes me study. When she does, I do some of my schoolwork. We argue a lot. If I sit alone in class and have no one to talk to I wouldn't interrupt so much, but I'm tempted to sit by my friends and talk. When I go out (from class) for a few minutes it helps me a little to calm down".

In the intervention process, in order to foster adaptive awareness, Ron's strengths were discussed first. Ron was aware of many of his assets, for example his talents for basketball, his good social skills and his intelligence. During treatment sessions, his understanding of strength areas expanded. Ron became aware of his good language skills through investigating of his psycho-educational evaluation. In addition Ron's good memory, learning abilities and flexibility in problem solving were uncovered through cognitive games. Ron's communication skills, his ability to express his thoughts and emotions and his ability to cooperate, were discovered through collaborative analysis of his interactions in the therapeutic context. Ron then identified the things that are important for him based on analyzing the manifestations of PVQ in daily life: to succeed in basketball and in school, to engage in fun activities, to care for his family and friends and to be able to listen to and accept their opinions, to have interests and challenges and to be independent. Following the psycho education unit regarding ADHD was introduced: Ron watched videos and presentations containing explanations and personal stories, and was asked which symptoms resemble his own. Ron acknowledged some of his challenges: "I am impulsive in school, I respond to everything being said in class. I interrupt my friends as they speak, and I can do dangerous stuff. It is hard for me to control my emotions; if something makes me angry I respond immediately and burst out. I'm disorganized in my schoolwork and it is very hard for me to recruit effort for studying". In the next sessions, Ron engaged in cognitive tasks and games that challenged inhibition, planning and recruiting effort. Ron was taught a task monitoring strategy that helped him gain a deeper understanding of his challenges "I don't stop and think before I start, I don't plan in advance". He started generating and practicing specific self-verbalization strategies 'stop is this good for me?' verbalize task steps in advance.

These discoveries led to Ron's formulation of his goal: 'to succeed in school'. Following, he was guided to define more specific and attainable goals and defined: 'not interrupting classes; 'prepare for tests' (see table C3). Ron chose to focus first on his first goal. Through applying the task analysis strategy he realized that 'not interrupting class requirements differ according to the teacher and that in classes with strict teachers (especially his math and science teachers) he can't talk at all. Ron decided to narrow his goal to 'not interrupting at all in classes with strict teachers" (math and science)'. Then, Ron analyzed which of his personal challenges might prevent him from achieving his goal: "my impulsiveness, I don't stop and think before I interrupt". Ron further analyzed the barriers in his environment: "other student talks to me, the teacher doesn't give me a warning before kicking me out of class". Ron also recognized some resources that may help: "I have good friends in my class, my teachers want me to succeed, I know the rules in my classroom, I have good communication skills, and I don't give up". Based on this awareness, Ron was able to generate strategies: "ask my friends not to talk to me during class", "ask permission to leave the classroom for a few minutes when I think I'm about to interrupt". Then Ron wrote his plan "when I feel I can't control myself, I will ask permission to go out for five minutes, get some air, relax and come back". A week later Ron reviewed his plan "it didn't work, I didn't feel I was interrupting and the teacher told me to go out for the whole lesson, I'm not sure why". This monitoring led to Ron to understand his difficulty with online awareness; "I don't notice when my behavior is problematic". Ron decided to ask his teachers for help, he wrote a new plan "I will talk with my teachers about my problem, and ask them to give me a sign whenever they think I am about to interrupt, then I will go out for five minutes". The next week Ron declared "this time my plan worked, my teachers agreed to help me, they signaled me, I went out and came back, I didn't interrupt. I know how to talk to people, I can persuade people to help me and signal me to control my behavior".

To foster social support, Ron's parents' guidance focused on understanding Ron's executive challenges and relating them to his ADHD. For example they understood that Ron's impulsiveness and poor emotional control may explain why discussions usually turn into arguments. They learned to adapt the way they discussed school work and domestic tasks by setting in advance, weekly discussion times when they are calm and able to collaborate well. They learned to provide nonjudgmental feedback and to ignore some of Ron's provocations. Following, Ron's parents were able to set more realistic goals for him. For example, the parents shifted their initial expectations that Ron will 'perform domestic tasks upon request' to 'perform domestic tasks that were set in the weekly discussion'.

The summary unit was an opportunity for Ron to consolidate his new learning. He prepared a video presentation of his process in therapy. He was very enthusiastic preparing this project. His presentation demonstrated improved awareness to his impulsiveness in many aspects of his life he also conveyed confidence in his ability to use resources to achieve occupational goals that were significant to him. His parents appeared to appreciate the steps he was taking along with his hard work. The family discussed the next steps to transfer these gains to their day-to-day life.

Table C1. BRIEF parent profile

Executive Function	T score pre*	T score post*
Inhibit	69	66
Shift	76	65
Emotional control	72	63
Initiate	63	59
Working memory	87	79
Plan/organize	74	59
Organization of materials	72	58
Monitor	82	57
Behavior Regulation Index	75	66
Meta cognitive Index	79	64
Global Executive	81	66

* (>65 considered deficient)

Table C2. Parent's COPM

Goal	Performance Pre (1-10)	Performance Post (1-10)
Accepts help in schoolwork	1	9
Study for tests	2	8
Perform domestic tasks that were set in in the weekly discussion	1	5. 5
More involvement with family	2	6

Table C3. Ron's COPM

Goal	Performance Pre (1-10)	Performance Post (1-10)
Not interrupting at all in classes with strict teachers	2. 5	8
Be prepared for tests	5. 5	8

Following intervention Ron and his parents reported clinically significant improvement (> 2 points on the COPM) in targeted goals (see tables C2 & C3). The parents ratings on the BRIEF also indicated a clinically significant improvement, with post-treatment scores below the impaired cutoff score (65) in emotional control, plan/organize, organization of materials, monitor and the Meta cognitive Index. Several scores still remained in the clinically impaired range (See table C1).

Case Studies Summary

Ron and Sara are facing multiple difficulties in their everyday functioning due to their executive dysfunction. They both experience a gap between their abilities and the requirements of their roles as students and family members. Sara is also struggling with social relationships. Both of them face recurrent negative feedback from their environment but lack understanding of their difficulties.

The intervention process demonstrates the enabling factors used in the Teen Cog-fun to help adolescents like Ron and Sara to bridge the gap between their abilities and the requirements of their roles. *Adaptive awareness* is targeted first. Through analysis of their occupational profile, experiences with cognitive tasks and games and guided learning of informational resources Ron and Sara gained insight. First they learned more about their strengths, then, they explored their values, and started facing their challenges. Facing challenges was accompanied with generating and practicing *cognitive strategies* that enabled them to envision overcoming them. This awareness set the stage for Ron and Sara to define their *occupational goals* that ware congruent with their personal profiles. Ron and Sara generated strategies and wrote plans to achieve their goals and were guided to review and analyze their experience in executing their plans. They discovered additional personal strengths and challenges, and environmental resources and barriers. Based on this knowledge they were able to adjust their strategies and refine their plans. In this process they learned global and specific executive strategies. Both sets of parents learned to better *support* their teens toward adaptive functioning with ADHD.

SUMMARY AND CONCLUSION

Adolescents with ADHD face an imbalance between demands and resources, thus they experience increasing challenges and recurrent failures. Intervention programs are needed in order to help adolescents with ADHD cope with their challenges, minimize risks and promote their options for an adaptive, productive life as adults. The Teen Cog-Fun is a psychosocial, integrative OT practice model that is designed to enable adolescents cope effectively with ADHD in their occupational contexts. The teen cog-fun protocol aims to support the development of *adaptive self-awareness, cognitive strategies and enabling environments* in order to promote satisfying participation in life roles and quality of life for the adolescents and their families. The Teen Cog-Fun principles and treatment methods are based on established OT and cognitive rehabilitation models. The MOHO (Kielhofner, 2008) provides the overarching framework, explaining the link between volition and occupation, and clarifies the importance of *enabling environments*; the BPS (Ownsworth et al., 2006) guides the treatment methods that target the development of *Adaptive self-awareness*; and the MTA (Toglia, 2011) guides the treatment methods for the development of *cognitive strategies* in occupational context. The standardized Teen Cog Fun treatment protocol forms a basis for examining the efficacy of this intervention in controlled trials.

REFERENCES

American Psychiatric Association (APA). (2000). *DSM: Diagnostic and statistical manual of mental disorders* (4[th]ed.). Washington DC: American Psychiatric Association.

Barbaresi, W., Katusic, S., Colligan, R., Weaver, A., & Jacobsen, S. (2007). Long-term school outcomes for children with attention-deficit/hyperactivity disorder: A population-based perspective. *Journal of Developmental and Behavioral Pediatrics, 28,* 265–273.

Barkley, R. A. (2006). *Attention-deficit hyperactivity disorder: A handbook for diagnosis and Treatment* (3[rd]ed.). New York, NY: Guilford Press.

Barkley, R. A. (2012). *Executive functions: What they are, how they work, and why they evolved,* New York, NY: Guilford Press.

Barkley, R. A., Fischer, M., Smallish, L., & Fletcher, K. (2006). Young Adult Outcome of Hyperactive Children: Adaptive Functioning in Major Life Activities. *Journal of American Academy of Child and Adolescents Psychiatry,* 45,192-202.

Barkley, R. A., & Cox, D. (2007). A review of driving risks and impairments associated with attention-deficit/hyperactivity disorder and the effects of stimulant medication on driving performance. *Journal of Safety Research,* 38, 113-128.

Biederman, J., Monuteaux, M. C. , Doyle, A. E. , Seidman, L. , J. , Wilens, T. E. , Ferrero, F., & Faraone, S. V. (2004). Impact of executive function deficits and Attention-Deficit/Hyperactivity Disorder (ADHD) on academic outcomes in children. *Journal of Consulting and Clinical Psychology, 72,* 757-766.

Biederman, J., Petty, C. R., Evans, M., Small, J., & Faraone, S. V. (2010). How persistent is ADHD? A controlled 10-year follow-up study of boys with ADHD. *Psychiatry Research,* 177, 299–304.

Brown, T. E. (2006). Executive functions and Attention Deficit Hyperactivity Disorder: Implications of two conflicting views. *International Journal of Disability, Development and Education.* 53, 35–46.

Brown, T. E. (2009). ADD/ADHD and Impaired Executive Function in Clinical Practice. *Current Attention Disorder Reports, 1,* 37-41.

Brown, T. E. (2013). *A new understanding of ADHD in children and adults: Executive function impairments.* New York, NY: Routledge.

Bussing, R., Koro-Ljungberg, M., Noguchi, K., Mason, D., Mayerson, G., & Garvan, C. W. (2012). Willingness to use ADHD treatments: A mixed methods study of perceptions by adolescents, parents, health professionals and teachers. *Social Science & Medicine, 74,* 92-100.

De Goede, I. H. A., Branje, S. J. T., & Meeus, W. H. J. (2009). Developmental changes in adolescents' perceptions of relationships with their parents. *Journal of Youth and Adolescence,* 38, 75–88.

Danckaerts, M., Heptinstall, E., Chadwick, O., &Taylor, E. (1999). Self-report of attention deficit and hyperactivity disorder in adolescents. *Psychopathology, 32,*91–92.

Edwards, G. , Barkley, R. , Laneri, M., Fletcher, K. , & Metevia, L. (2001). Parent–adolescent conflict in teenagers with ADHD and ODD. *Journal of Abnormal Child Psychology, 29,* 557–572.

Elkins, I. J. , McGue, M. , & Iacono, W. G. (2007). Prospective effects of attention-deficit/hyperactivity disorder, conduct disorder, and sex on adolescent substance use and abuse. *Archives of General Psychiatry, 64,* 1145-1152.

Flory, K., Molina, B., Pelham, W., Gnagy, E., & Smith, B. (2006). Childhood ADHD predicts risky sexual behavior in young adulthood. *Journal of Clinical Child and Adolescent Psychology, 35,* 571–577.

Frazier, T. W., Youngstrom, E. A., Glutting, J. J, & Watkins, M. W. (2007). ADHD and achievement: meta-analysis of the child, adolescent, and adult literatures and a concomitant study with college students. *Journal of Learning Disabilities, 40,* 49-65.

Geissler, J., & Lesch, K. P. (2011). A lifetime of attention-deficit/hyperactivity disorder: diagnostic challenges, treatment and neurobiological mechanisms. *Expert Review of Neurotherapeutics,* 11, 1467-1484.

Gioia, G. A., Isquith, P. K., Guy, S. C., & Kenworthy, L. (2000a). *Behavior Rating Inventory of Executive Function (BRIEF).* Odessa, FL: Psychological Assessment Resources.

Glatz, T., Stattin, H., & Kerr, M. (2011). Parents' reactions to youths' hyperactivity, impulsivity, and attention problems. *Journal of Abnormal Child Psychology, 39,* 1125–1135.

Gudjonsson, G. H. Sigurdsson, J. F., Sigfusdottir, I. D., & Young, S. (2012). An epidemiological study of ADHD symptoms among young persons and the relationship with cigarette smoking, alcohol consumption and illicit drug use. *Journal of Child Psychology and Psychiatry, 53,*304–312.

Katz, N., & Maeir, A. (2011). Higher-Level Cognitive Functions Enabling Participation: Awareness and Executive Functions. In N. Katz (Ed.). Cognition, Occupation, and Participation across the Life Span: Neuroscience, *Neurorehabilitation, and Models of Intervention in Occupational Therapy, 3rd Ed.* (pp. 13-40). Bethesda, MD:AOTA Press.

Kielhofner, G. (2008). *Model of Human Occupation: Theory and Application* (4th ed.). Baltimore: Lippincott Williams & Wilkins.

Kortte, K. B., & Wegener, T. (2004). Denial of illness in medical rehabilitation populations: Theory, research and definition. *Rehabilitation Psychology, 49,* 187-199.

Law, M., Baptiste, S., Carswell, A., McColl, M. A., Polataijko, H., & Pollock, N. (2005). *The Canadian Occupational Performance Measure (3rd Edition).* Toronto, ON: COAT.

Lifford, K. J., Harold, G. T., & Thapar, A. (2008). Parent-child relationships and ADHD symptoms: a longitudinal analysis. *Journal of Abnormal Child Psychology, 36,* 285–296.

Lifford, K. J., Harold, G. T., & Thapar, A. (2009). Parent-child hostility and child ADHD symptoms: a genetically sensitive and longitudinal analysis. *Journal of Child Psychology and Psychiatry, 50,* 1468–1476.

Murray-Close, D., Hoza, B. , Hinshaw, S. P., Arnold, L. E., Swanson, J., Jensen, P. S. Wells, K. (2010). Developmental processes in peer problems of children with attention-deficit/hyperactivity disorder in the Multimodal Treatment Study of children with ADHD: Developmental cascades and vicious cycles. *Development and Psychopathology, 22,* 785–802.

National Institute for Health and Clinical Excellence. (2008). *Attention deficit hyperactivity disorder: Diagnosis and management of ADHD in children, young people and adults.* www. nice. org. uk

National Institute of Mental Health. (2008). *Attention Deficit Hyperactivity Disorder (ADHD).* nimh. nih. gov

Ownsworth, T., Clare, L., & Morris, R. (2006). An integrated biopsychosocial approach to understanding awareness deficits in Alzheimer's disease and brain injury. *Neuropsychological Rehabilitation, 16,* 415-438.

Roley, S. S., DeLany, J. V., Barrows, C. J., Brownrigg, S., Honaker, D., Sava, D. I., ... & Youngstrom, M. J. (2008). Occupational therapy practice framework: domain & practice. *The American journal of Occupational Therapy 62,* (6), 625.

Rubin, K. H., Bukowski, W. M., & Parker, J. G. (2006). Peer interactions, relationships, and groups. In N. Eisenberg, W. Damon & R. M. Lerner (Eds.), *Handbook of child psychology: Social, emotional, and personality development*6th ed. pp. 571–645. Hoboken: Wiley.

Schwartz, S. H. (1992). Universals in the content and structure of values: Theory and empirical tests in 20 countries. In M. Zanna (Ed.), *Advances in experimental social psychology (Vol. 25)* (pp. 1-65). New York: Academic Press.

Schwartz, S. H., Melech, G., Lehmann, A., Burgess, S., & Harris, M. (2001). Extending the cross-cultural validity of the theory of basic human values with a different method of measurement. *Journal of Cross-Cultural Psychology, 32,* 519-542.

Sibley, M. H., Evans, S. W., &. Serpell, Z. N. (2010). Social cognition and interpersonal impairment in young adolescents with ADHD. *Journal ofPsychopathology and Behavioral Assessment,* 32, 193–202.

Sibley, M. H., Pelham, W. E., Molina, B. S. G., Gnagy, E. M., Waschbusch, D. A. , Biswas, A., Karch, K. (2011). The delinquency outcomes of boys with ADHD with and without comorbidity. *Journal of Abnormal Child Psychology, 39,* 21–32.

Sibley, M. H., Pelham, W. E., Molina, B. S. G., Gnagy, E. M., Waschbusch, D. A., Garefino, Karch, K. M. (2012). Diagnosing ADHD in adolescence. *Journal of Consulting and Clinical Psychology*, 80, 139-150.

Smith, B. H., Waschbusch, D. A., Willoughby, M. T., & Evans, S. (2000). The efficacy, safety, and practicality of treatments for adolescents with Attention-Deficit/Hyperactivity Disorder (ADHD). *Clinical Child and Family Psychology Review, 3,* 243-267.

Turgay, A., Goodman, D. W. Asherson, P., Lasser, R. A., Babcock, T. F, Pucci. M. L., Barkley, R. ADHD Transition Phase Model Working Group. (2012). Lifespan persistence of ADHD: The life transition model and its application. *Journal of Clinical Psychiatry*, 73(2), 192-201.

Toglia, J. P. (2011). The dynamic interactional model of cognition in cognitive rehabilitation. In N. Katz (Ed.), Cognition, Occupation, and Participation across the Life Span: Neuroscience, *Neurorehabilitation, and Models of Intervention in Occupational Therapy, 3rd Ed.* (pp. 161-201). Bethesda, MD:AOTA Press.

Toglia, J., & Kirk, U. (2000). Understanding awareness deficits following brain injury. *NeuroRehabilitation, 15,* 57–70.

Volz-Sidiropoulou, E., Boecker, M., & Gauggel, S. (in press). The Positive Illusory Bias in children and adolescents with ADHD: Further evidence. *Journal of Attention Disorders.*

Wilens, T. E., Martelon, M. K., Joshi, G., Bateman, C., Fried, R. , Pctty, C. , & Biederman, J. (2011). Does ADHD predict substance-use disorders? A 10-year follow-up study of young adults with ADHD. *Journal Of The American Academy Of Child & Adolescent Psychiatry,50 ,* 543-553.

Willcutt, E. G., Doyle, A. E., Nigg, J. T., Faraone, S. V., & Pennington, B. F. (2005). Validity of the executive function theory of Deficit/Hyperactivity Disorder: A meta-analytic review. *Biological Psychiatry*, 57, 1336-1346.

World Health Organization. (2001). *International classification of functioning, disability and health.* Geneva: World Health Organization.

Yoshimasu, K., Barbaresi, W. J., Colligan, R. C., Voigt, R. G., Killian, J. M., Weaver, A. L. & Katusic, S. K. (2012). Childhood ADHD is strongly associated with a broad range of psychiatric disorders during adolescence: a population-based birth cohort study. *Journal of Child Psychology and Psychiatry, 53,* 1036–1043.

Young, S., Gudjonsson, G., Misch, P., Collins, P., Carter, P., Redfern, J. & Goodwin, E (2010). Prevalence of ADHD symptoms among youth in a secure facility: the consistency and accuracy of self- and informant-report ratings. *The Journal of Forensic Psychiatry & Psychology, 21,* 238–246.

In: ADHD
Editors: Itai Berger and Adina Maeir

ISBN: 978-1-63321-047-9
© 2014 Nova Science Publishers, Inc.

Chapter 3

GIFTEDNESS AND ADHD

Iris Manor, M.D. *

Geha Mental Health Center, Petach-Tiqva, Israel

ABSTRACT

Gifted children with ADHD do suffer from executive dysfunctions, be they compensated or un-compensated by the giftedness. Their suffering, from the outer as well as from the inner perspective is real, and their development might well be harmed.

This chapter described the complicated issues of diagnosis and treatment of ADHD in gifted children.

Gifted children deserve, as all others, the best treatment they can get, but in this special group it should be planned for both aspects of their "twice exceptionality".

GIFTEDNESS

Giftedness is more than a number, more than a better score in tests. It is the ability to understand things "from thin air", a very rapid and associative-like way of thought. While studies regarding gifted children and adolescents exist, they are mostly concerned with cognitive abilities, psychometric characteristics and the best way to help their development.

Surprisingly, there are very few psychiatric studies dealing with giftedness, their psychodynamic status, the frequency of different comorbidities with giftedness and their inner perceptions.

In recent decades research in the literature regarding giftedness has shifted from focusing on who the gifted are to how the gifted think [1]. It is known that gifted children differ from their average-ability peers as they have a broader knowledge base and are more capable of using that knowledge to their benefit; they prefer complex, challenging environments; they are quicker at solving problems but spend more time in the solution planning stage; they represent and categorize problems more efficiently; they have finely tuned procedural know-

---

* Corresponding author: Iris Manor, M.D. Child and adolescent Psychiatrist. Director of ADHD Unit, Geha Mental Health Center, Petach-Tiqva, Israel. E-mail: IManor@clalit.org.il.

ledge; they are flexible in their strategies and problem solutions, and they are more sophisticated in their meta-cognition and self-regulation. Many studies deal with these abilities, but since they are not the scope of this chapter, they will not be dealt with now.

When crossing the border from the intellectual to the emotional field, knowledge becomes sparse. Gifted people suffer and suffered from many stigma and are prone to be ambivalently looked upon. On one hand the giftedness itself is a source of respect and even envy, on the other hand gifted people are considered immature, socially dysfunctional and more. A good example of this ambivalence is demonstrated in the movie (based on the play) Amadeus. Mozart is the genius, but he is also the petty child.

But is this the real clinical picture?

Development is usually described as moving along three main axles: biological – growth, hormonal; psychological – cognitive and mental; and social. In order to have a harmonic development, the rate of all three has to be similar, more or less. For example, a normal child at the age of six years has to have the height and the weight of a six year old, cognitively, if he is intelligent six and a half, mentally around six and a half years and socially quite the same. A gifted child of the same age group will have the same developmental characteristics, except for one: cognitively he will be at the age of 9-10 years old. Many times the mental state may be influenced and it will also be higher than expected. But, this development is disharmonious, or as it is called by Goerss [2] "asynchronous development", meaning that the gap between the cognitive aspects and the others might create an illusion of immaturity. This might happen because the environment, as well as the child himself or herself will judge his/her behavior according to the standards of an older age groups, as is almost inevitable because of his/her cognitive abilities and his/her way of thinking. This gap is confusing, and many times leads to mistaken expectations hence mistaken judgment. This gap gets bigger when the child (as it happens many times) is put in a class of older children because of his/her advanced cognitive abilities. Another explanation of this difficult social development, made by Goerss, is that the social environment is not "tailored enough" to the gifted child. The sociological demand requested during childhood is identifying with your peers. The gifted child, according to Goerss, has difficulty in this task, because of different ways of thoughts and areas of interest.

Accordingly, the normal social development is disturbed, not because of an immaturity of the gifted child, but because of his/her asynchrony with his/her social environment.

Another characteristic of gifted children is their huge curiosity, which is frequently accompanied by a lot of imagination and high sensitivity. This characteristic causes gifted children to reach places which are not accommodated to their mental age: hearing news, reading non-fiction books, analyzing situations all of which are too advanced for them and scare them. It could be illustrated to a cat that climbs on a tree too high to get down by itself.

The result of all these characteristics is that these children are many time self-critical and self-disappointed, which increases the illusion of emotionally disturbed children.

Interestingly, in a study by Field et al. [3], the differences between the self-perceptions of gifted high school freshmen and non-gifted peers were assessed. It was found, that the gifted students were socially precocious. They also perceived themselves as the same or better than their peers about their academic and social skills, but, their teachers rated them as being less happy than their peers (Field, 1998). It seems that in contrast to the common views, these children are precocious not only in their academic capabilities but also in their social ones.

What happens in the emotional world of the gifted child? Lind [4] claims that intensity, sensitivity and over-excitability are primary characteristics of gifted children, but this suggestion is based mainly on naturalistic observations and much less on evidence-based studies. She quoted the Polish psychiatrist and psychologist, Dabrowski, who believed in "positive disintegration" in which inner suffering and conflict are essential for advanced development [5]. In an appendix [6], results of studies with a group of gifted children and young people were described. Dabrowski [6] found that every one of the gifted children displayed over-excitability. He suggested that the cause "is more than average sensitivity which not only permits one to achieve outstanding results in learning and work, but at the same time increases the number of points sensitive to all experiences that may accelerate anomalous reactions revealing themselves in psychoneurotic sets". This association between over-excitability and giftedness was also shown in other studies [7, 8]. These studies suggest that over-excitability is at least one of the markers of potential for giftedness/creativity.

ADHD

ADHD is a disorder, in which there are several executive dysfunctions, specific clinical symptoms of inattention, hyperactivity and impulsivity, and dysregulations in different biological rhythms. The most recent edition of the DSM, DSM-5 has re-defined some important concepts about ADHD, the most important one is its being now considered a neuro-developmental disorder and not a disruptive behavior disorder [9].

The concept of ADHD as a neuro-developmental disorder is strengthened and widened by Gillberg [10] as he terms a new concept, the ESSENCE. The acronym ESSENCE refers to Early Symptomatic Syndromes Eliciting Neurodevelopmental Clinical Examinations and refers to a co-existence of disorders - including ADHD, oppositional defiant disorder, tic disorder, developmental coordination disorder, and autism spectrum disorder. According to Gillberg [10], sharing of symptoms across disorders (sometimes referred to as comorbidity) is the rule rather than the exception in child psychiatry and developmental medicine. Gillberg does not include exceptional intelligence as one of the ESSENCE components, but it seems that some characteristics of giftedness and ADHD are shared nevertheless.

In this chapter I will examine the relationships between giftedness and ADHD symptom-matology. I will discuss in detail the empirical studies in this field, the relationships between cognitive functioning and ADHD symptomatology, the implications for unique diagnostic demands in this group, the validity of ADHD diagnosis in the high IQ/giftedness population with comparisons to average IQ ADHD, educational implications, the effects of medications on creativity, and the implications for future studies in the field.

CLINICAL ISSUES

The diagnosis of ADHD in children with a high intellectual quotient (IQ)/giftedness is controversial. Over the past 20 years, there has been considerable debate over the validity of an ADHD diagnosis in this group.

It is also a neglected issue, and despite many existing opinions, very few empirical data have reported scientific results asserting the validity of ADHD in the specific population [11].

Interestingly, some of the empirical support for the importance of metacognition in giftedness comes from the study of learning-disabled gifted students [1]. In their review, they showed that although metacognitive deficits are considered at least partially responsible for learning problems, when giftedness and learning disabilities occur in the same individual, giftedness often "prevails" and metacognitive performance is only slightly affected. It should be noted however, that the studies quoted by Steiner and Carr did not separate ADHD from learning disabilities, and therefore we cannot be sure that the same rule applies to ADHD as well.

Clinical studies suggest that ADHD is difficult to diagnose in part because individuals with ADHD share characteristics, such as high energy and creativity, with gifted, non-ADHD individuals. Moreover, their very high intellectual ability tends to mask, at least up to a point, their executive dysfunctions. It seems, that in classical executive tests, the real-life executive functions deficits in the high functioning ADHD patients are not defined enough. In a recent study, high cognitive functioning adult ADHD participants were tested on standard and "highly demanding" executive tasks [12]. They found that compared to low functioning adults with ADHD, the high-functioning ones did not differ from the "healthy" control group. However, when they were tested on an "ecological" task of executive function (the hotel task) and computerized tasks of high cognitive demand, there was a significant dysfunction in the high-functioning group. The conclusions of the authors were that high-functioning adults with ADHD do suffer from executive dysfunctions, but these dysfunctions cannot be measured by the standard tests [12].

Another study terms ADHD and giftedness as "twice exceptional" [13]. The authors suggest that there is an overemphasis on a purely behavioral, categorical approach to understanding human function. This overemphasis, as they define it does not include a consideration of overlapping levels of function, hence neglects several comorbidities, which could be defined only by the corticocentric model of function [13].

On the other hand, Antshel et al. [14] investigated the validity of ADHD in high IQ children compared to "healthy" high IQ children. This longitudinal family study compared the clinical characteristics of high IQ children with and without ADHD and those of their families. It was found that the majority of children with ADHD and a high IQ, met criteria for the combined subtype. These children when compared to control participants had a higher prevalence of familial ADHD in first-degree relatives.

They also showed the same clinical characteristics demonstrated by average IQ children with ADHD, i.e., they repeated grades more often, had a poorer performance on the WISC-III Block Design, had more comorbid psychopathology, and had more functional impairments across a number of domains. These results suggest that giftedness does not protect children with ADHD from the executive dysfunctions of the disorder, and their familial cognitive, psychiatric and behavioral features do not differ from the general population of children with ADHD [14].

A study by Brown et al. [15] demonstrated quite the same thing and even further than that; high IQ children and adolescents diagnosed with ADHD tend to suffer from executive function (EF) impairments. The EF impairments could be identified with a combination of standardized measures and normed self-report data, and occurred even more frequently in this group than in the general population [15].

Another study, [16] asked the same questions, testing the strategic verbal memory processes among intellectually gifted youth with and without ADHD, however reached a different conclusion. While it was found that the intellectually gifted youth with ADHD achieved significantly lower T scores compared with intellectually gifted youth without ADHD, they achieved higher T scores than youth of average intellectual abilities with ADHD. Additionally, gifted youth with ADHD showed a main effect improvement in short-delay recall when provided with organizational cues [16].

COMPARISON

Another interesting point to discuss is the high similarity between some of the ADHD characteristics and these of giftedness. Either feature, or syndrome, tend to be extreme and to be demonstrated by extreme behaviors. They are both hereditary [17, 18].

They are not always easy to be seen, which causes many doubts, both by the environment and by the person himself. Both are considered to be more frequent in boys than in girls, and both tend to be highly stigmatized.

These similarities are not only interesting, but theoretically may imply that extreme intelligence may be part of ESSENCE as well.

SUMMARY OF THE CLINICAL PICTURE

In summary, giftedness does not protect one from executive dysfunction, but rather masks it. It has two contradicting facets: being "twice exceptional" which highlights the differences between the gifted child with ADHD and others [13], and the masking of the executive dysfunctions by the giftedness [14]. It should also be kept in mind that the clinical picture of the gifted child with ADHD is usually twice masked, as well as paradoxical. This paradox is big enough that even the possibility of a protecting effect of being gifted on the executive dysfunctions is not agreed upon [14, 15].

Hence, this masking goes both ways, since the ADHD is masked by the giftedness, but many times the giftedness, especially when it is tested using "regular" tests, is masked by the ADHD. Either way, the gifted child with ADHD is even more clinically exceptional than the normal child with ADHD or the gifted child without ADHD, and is a bigger challenge to the clinician, who faces a much more complex picture, which is worth a discussion by itself.

Clinically speaking, from the outside, this "twice exception" might become "twice extreme". The differences between the gifted child with ADHD and his/her peers become bigger and more confusing. For instance, it could be the same child who solves the most complex problems at class, becomes bored and doesn't have enough common interests with his/her peers. At the same time, this child might fail in much easier tasks, be clumsy and forgetful, and demonstrate significant executive function deficits. How would such a child be understood? Many times these children are considered spoiled, arrogant or neglectful, or they might be seen only through the prism of their difficulties, ignoring their special abilities.

From the inside, gifted children with ADHD have very similar paradoxes to solve. They too are confused because of the significant difference among their abilities.

This confusion might result in self-criticism ("what an idiot I am that I couldn't do this simple task, and children much more stupid than I managed it"), self-disappointment, and as a result, a very low self-esteem. These emotions lead many times to great anger, a feeling of impotency and a disintegrated sense of self; the variation between different self-images, revolving from different tasks, might lead to the impossibility of having one integrated self-image, but to the contrary, very different self-images (for example, great in math but failing in arithmetic) which prevent an integrated image on one's self.

Another dangerous way of thought is using their very high intellect as an excuse to dismiss treatment (specifically medications), claiming that these children could and should compensate, even if it means that they will be blocked from developing their unique abilities. This claim is "pseudo-logical", but it ignores the special needs of these children resulting from their giftedness. Hence, this claim results in "double damage", that is the ADHD will not be treated, and the giftedness will be neglected, including all the cognitive, social and emotional aspects related to it.

TREATMENT

How do we treat gifted children with ADHD? Should we treat them? One of the most frequent misconceptions is the belief that the giftedness will compensate for the executive dysfunctions of the ADHD, and even worse, that which leads to excluding gifted children with ADHD from activities intended to "regular" gifted children. One of the reasons of this belief may be the fear of medications. But what is really the effect of medications on gifted children? Is it different by any means?

Grizenko et al. [19], compared ADHD children with a borderline intelligence quotient (IQ) ($70{\leq}FSIQ{<}80$), normal IQ ($80{\leq}FSIQ{<}120$) and high IQ ($FSIQ{\geq}120$) according to their response to psycho-stimulants, the most common and most effective treatment of ADHD. No significant differences were found with regards to treatment response; the conclusion being that "proper medication management is necessary for all children with the disorder" [19].

Another question that exists is not directly about giftedness, but rather about its companion, creativity. Another common belief is that creativity is related to ADHD and thus may be harmed by ADHD medications.

In a 40-year prospective study about mental illness and creativity [20] Kyaga et al. asked if creativity was associated with all psychiatric disorders or was restricted to those with psychotic features. Creative professions were defined as scientific and artistic occupations. Except for bipolar disorder, individuals with overall creative professions were not more likely to suffer from investigated psychiatric disorders than controls, including ADHD. There was also no association between creative professions and first-degree relatives of patients with ADHD [20].

Healy and Rucklidge [21] studied the relationship between ADHD and creativity from the perspective of executive functions. They showed that 40% of the creative children in their sample displayed clinically elevated levels of ADHD symptomatology, but none met full criteria for ADHD. With regard to cognitive functioning, both ADHD and creative children with ADHD symptoms had deficits in naming speed, processing speed, and reaction time, meaning that creativity did not compensate for these dysfunctions.

On the other hand, in all other cognitive measures the creative group with ADHD symptoms outperformed the ADHD group. These findings have implications for the development and management of creative children [21].

There is only very scarce literature about this subject, but it seems that the treatment with medications does not result in any "damage to creativity" [22, 23]. Funk et al. [22] studied both the executive functions and the response to methylphenidate (MPH) in ADHD children, creative and not creative. They demonstrated that when measured nonverbally, the creative thinking performance of boys with ADHD was not superior to that of peers who did not have ADHD. Regarding the effects of MPH, prescribed therapy did not influence performance on this measure of creative thinking [22].

Farah et al. [23] studied the effects of Adderall on the performance of 16 healthy young adults as were measured on four tests of creativity: two tasks requiring divergent thought and two requiring convergent thought. They demonstrated that Adderall affected performance on the convergent tasks only, in one case enhancing it, particularly for lower-performing individuals, and in the other case enhancing it for the lower-performing and impairing it for higher-performing individuals. They concluded that opposite to the hypothesis that Adderall has an overall negative effect on creativity Its effects on convergent creative thought appear to be dependent on the baseline performance of the convergence ability of the individual. Those in the higher range of the normal distribution may be unaffected or impaired, whereas those in the lower range of the normal distribution experience enhancement.

This means that adults that suffer from executive dysfunction, resulting in impairment in convergent thought, will benefit from medication [23].

CONCLUSION

In summary, gifted children with ADHD do suffer from executive dysfunctions, be they compensated or un-compensated by the giftedness. Their suffering, from the outer as well as from the inner perspective is real, and their development might well be harmed.

Therefore gifted children deserve, as all children do, the best treatment they can get, but in this special group it should be planned for both aspects of their "twice exceptionality".

They should be treated for ADHD according to all the guidelines of the professional literature, meaning medications, psycho-education etc., and at the same time they should be referred to the same settings structured for all the gifted children in their community in order to help them achieve the most fitting and harmonious development.

REFERENCES

[1]   Steiner, H. H., Carr, M. Cognitive Development in Gifted Children: Toward a More Precise Understanding of Emerging Differences in Intelligence. *Educational Psychology Review*, Vol. 15, No. 3, September 2003.

[2]   Goerss, J. Asynchronous development. Part II: Understanding giftedness. In: *Supporting Emotional needs of the Gifted: 30 years of Giftedness, 30 years of SENG.*

By Supporting Emotional Needs of the Gifted (Author), SENG Authors September 2012, SENG. POB 488, Poughquag, NY 12570.

[3] Field, T., Harding, J., Yando, R., Gonzalez, K., Lasko, D., Bendell, D., Marks, C. *Feelings and attitudes of gifted students Adolescence.* 1998 Summer; 33(130):331-42.

[4] Lind, S. Overexcitability and the gifted. In: Part II: Understanding giftedness, In: *Supporting Emotional needs of the Gifted: 30 years of Giftedness, 30 years of SENG.* By Supporting Emotional Needs of the Gifted (Author), SENG Authors September 2012, SENG. POB 488, Poughquag, NY 12570.

[5] Dąbrowski, K. (1966). "The Theory of Positive Disintegration". *International Journal of Psychiatry* 2: 229–44.

[6] Dąbrowski, K. (1967). *Personality-shaping through Positive Disintegration.* Boston, Mass.: Little Brown.

[7] Piechowski, M. M. (1986). "The Concept of Developmental Potential". *Roeper Review* 8 (3): 190–97.

[8] Piechowski, M. M., Miller, N. B. (1995). "Assessing Developmental Potential in Gifted Children: A Comparison of Methods". *Roeper Review* 17 (3): 176–80.

[9] Dalsgaard, S. Attention-deficit/hyperactivity disorder (ADHD). *Eur. Child Adolesc. Psychiatry.* 2013 Feb.;22 Suppl. 1:S43-8.

[10] Gillberg, C. The ESSENCE in child psychiatry: Early Symptomatic Syndromes Eliciting Neurodevelopmental Clinical Examinations. *Res. Dev. Disabil.* 2010 Nov.-Dec.;31(6):1543-51.

[11] Antshel, K. M. Attention-Deficit Hyperactivity Disorder in the context of a high intellectual quotient/giftedness. *Dev. Disabil. Res. Rev.* 2008;14(4):293-9.

[12] Torralva, T., Gleichgerrcht, E., Lischinsky, A., Roca, M., Manes, F. Ecological" and Highly Demanding Executive Tasks Detect Real-Life Deficits in High-Functioning Adult ADHD Patients. *J. Atten. Disord.* 2012 Jul. 23.

[13] Budding, D., Chidekel, D. ADHD and giftedness: a neurocognitive consideration of twice exceptionality. *Appl. Neuropsychol. Child.* 2012;1(2):145-51.

[14] Antshel, K. M., Faraone, S. V., Stallone, K., Nave, A., Kaufmann, F. A., Doyle, A., Fried, R., Seidman, L., Biederman, J. Is attention deficit hyperactivity disorder a valid diagnosis in the presence of high IQ? Results from the MGH Longitudinal Family Studies of ADHD. *J. Child Psychol. Psychiatry.* 2007 Jul.;48(7):687-94.

[15] Brown, T. E., Reichel, F. C., Quinlan, D. M. Executive function impairments in high IQ children and adolescents with ADHD. *Open Journal of Psychiatry*, 2011, 1, 56-65.

[16] Whitaker, A. M., Bell, T. S., Houskamp, B. M., O'Callaghan, E. T. A Neurodevelopmental approach to understanding memory processes among intellectually gifted youth with Attention-Deficit Hyperactivity Disorder. *Appl. Neuropsychol. Child.* 2013 Nov. 5.

[17] Oerter, R. Biological and psychological correlates of exceptional performance in development. *Ann. N. Y. Acad. Sci.* 2003 Nov.; 999:451-60.

[18] Akutagava-Martins, G. C. 1, Salatino-Oliveira, A., Kieling, C. C., Rohde, L. A., Hutz, M. H. Genetics of attention-deficit/hyperactivity disorder: current findings and future directions. *Expert Rev. Neurother.* 2013 Apr.;13(4):435-45.

[19] Grizenko, N., Qi Zhang, D. D., Polotskaia, A., Joober, R. Efficacy of methylphenidate in ADHD children across the normal and the gifted intellectual spectrum. *J. Can. Acad. Child Adolesc. Psychiatry.* 2012 Nov.;21(4):282-8.

[20] Kyaga, S., Landén, M., Boman, M., Hultman, C. M., Långström, N., Lichtenstein, P. Mental illness, suicide and creativity: 40-year prospective total population study. *J. Psychiatr. Res.* 2013 Jan.;47(1):83-90.

[21] Healey, D., Rucklidge, J. J. An investigation into the relationship among ADHD symptomatology, creativity, and neuropsychological functioning in children. *Child Neuropsychol.* 2006 Dec.;12(6):421-38.

[22] Funk, J. B., Chessare, J. B., Weaver, M. T., Exley, A. R. Attention deficit hyperactivity disorder, creativity, and the effects of methylphenidate. *Pediatrics.* 1993 Apr.;91(4): 816-9.

[23] Farah, M. J., Haimm, C., Sankoorikal, G., Smith, M. E., Chatterjee, A. When we enhance cognition with Adderall, do we sacrifice creativity? A preliminary study. *Psychopharmacology* (Berl.). 2009 Jan.; 202(1-3):541-7.

In: ADHD

ISBN: 978-1-63321-047-9

Editors: Itai Berger and Adina Maeir

© 2014 Nova Science Publishers, Inc.

Chapter 4

THE RELATIONSHIP BETWEEN ADHD AND SMD

*Aviva Yochman, Ph.D.** and Tal Mazor-Karsenty*

School of Occupational Therapy, Hadassah and
Hebrew University, Mount Scopus, Jerusalem, Israel

ABSTRACT

Attention Deficit Hyperactivity Disorder (ADHD) is among the most prevalent and widely researched of childhood disorders. Its adverse effect on multiple areas of a child's daily functioning has major implications for these children and their families, as well as for society as a whole. However, apart from the core deficits of the disorder, ADHD is often associated with various co-existing neuro-developmental impairments, among them, Sensory Modulation Disorder (SMD). While research focusing on the relationship between ADHD and SMD is relatively new, it has been receiving increasing attention in recent years.

In view of the wide-ranging influence that sensory modulation has on daily functioning and quality of life, it is imperative that clinicians working with children with ADHD become familiar with this research and its significant implications for this population.

This chapter will provide a short summary of the salient characteristics of both ADHD and SMD, followed by a summary of the literature regarding the relationship between the two disorders. A discussion of the theoretical and clinical implications will then follow.

ATTENTION DEFICIT HYPERACTIVITY DISORDER

Attention deficit hyperactivity disorder (ADHD) is characterized by inattention, hyper-activity, impulsivity, or a combination of these symptoms, to a degree which compromises everyday functioning (Feldman and Reiff, 2014).

---

* Corresponding author: Aviva Yochman, Ph.D. School of Occupational Therapy, Hadassah and Hebrew University, PO Box 24026, Mount Scopus, Jerusalem, 91240. E-mail: aviva.yochman@mail.huji.ac.il.

Attention problems are generally described as distractibility and difficulty in sustaining attention. Children with ADHD appear to be in constant motion. They have difficulty keeping their body still, displaying restlessness, fidgeting and excessive gross bodily movements. Their impulsivity manifests as an inability to withhold inappropriate responses, a tendency to respond prematurely, an excessive attraction to immediate rewards, as well as acting without reflection, recklessness and impetuous behavior (Cermak, 2005). Since both inattention and hyperactivity-impulsivity are multidimensional constructs, qualitatively different forms of impairments may eventually be found among these children (Barkley, 2003).

Although ADHD has traditionally been viewed as a problem relating to inattention and hyperactivity-impulsivity, current research indicates that ADHD is associated with prominent impairments of executive or higher order control functions (Barkley, 2003; Brown, 2013; Nigg, 2005).

In the majority of children, the effect of ADHD on functional performance is profound and widespread, affecting multiple developmental domains, including cognitive, academic, social, emotional and behavioral (Daley, 2005). According to the Diagnostic and Statistical Manual of Mental Disorders (DSM-5) there are three subtypes of the disorder: a) predominantly inattentive, b) predominantly hyperactive-impulsive, and c) combined type. For diagnostic criteria to be fulfilled the symptoms displayed should be clearly excessive in relation to the child's developmental level, must persist for at least 6 months, be observable in at least two settings (e.g., home and school) and at least some should have emerged before the age of 12. In addition, the symptoms should be such that they interfere with social, occupational or academic functioning (APA, 2013). Although it is well accepted that ADHD is heterogeneous in its presentation (Barkley, Murphy, and Kwasnik, 2006), not much neuroanatomic evidence exists validating these subtypes (Koziol and Budding, 2012). The DSM-5 (APA, 2013) states a prevalence of 5% among children in most cultures, with a ratio of 2 boys:1 girl in the general population.

ADHD follows a chronic course and accumulating evidence indicates that symptoms of ADHD persist into adulthood (Kessler, Green, Adeler et al., 2010). In adolescence and adulthood, ADHD has been associated with elevated rates of work and academic problems, lower occupational achievement, and increased risk for delinquency, substance abuse, anti-social behaviors and psychiatric disorders (Brown, 2013).

Due to the often pervasive effects of the disorder and its chronicity, treatment for both children and adults is multifaceted and generally prolonged (Dunn and Kronenberger, 2003).

The precise etiology of ADHD still remains unclear, although significant progress has been made in defining this area. The potentially causative factors associated with ADHD that have received the most research support are genetic and neuro-biological in nature (Nigg, 2005). Nevertheless, researchers acknowledge that the child's environment does play a role in the maintenance and severity of symptom development across time (Barkley, 2003; Morrell and Murray, 2003). In addition, and most importantly, researchers emphasize genetic-environmental correlations (Rutter and Silberg, 2002).

Studies indicate that it is unlikely that one single mechanism can account for the symptomatic heterogeneity of ADHD, the multi-factorial determined etiology, as well as the difficulty in differentiating ADHD from other childhood psychopathological disorders with similar behavioral features (Cermak, 2005; Nigg, 2005).

It is important to emphasize that ADHD is usually associated with additional difficulties than those subsumed under the ADHD diagnosis per se. Moreover, the nature and prevalence of co-occurring deficits in individuals with ADHD have recently come to the forefront as a highly important aspect of the disorder (Gillberg, Gillberg, Rasmussen, Kadesjo, Soderstrom, and Rastam, 2004). Both clinical (e.g., Conner, Edward, Fletcher, Baird, Barkley, and Steingard, 2003) and community studies (e.g., Kadesjo and Gillberg, 2001) have found extremely elevated rates of co-occurrence between ADHD and a wide variety of disorders. In addition, numerous studies have shown that most children, adolescents and adults who meet the diagnostic criteria for ADHD also meet the criteria for at least one additional disorder and some meet the criteria for several different disorders (Brown, 2013).

Several hypotheses have been advanced to try and explain the co-occurrence between ADHD and the various disorders. One possible argument is that ADHD and the co-existing disorder/s share a common etiology (Angold, Costello, and Erkanli, 1999; Gillberg et al., 2004). An alternative explanation relates to the possibility that there is a sequential relationship between the disorders, such that one disorder creates an increased risk for another (Denckla, 2003; Tseng, Henderson, Chow, and Yao, 2004).

Yet another explanation is that comorbidity is a result of two clearly distinct and separate disorders that may co-occur in the same individual but are unlinked either etiologically or sequentially (Angold et al., 1999; Gillberg et al., 2004). It has also been suggested that specific combinations of co-existing disorders may represent distinct subtypes within the ADHD spectrum with different clinical presentations, etiological factors, course and response to treatment (Brown, 2000; Jensen, Martin, and Cantwell, 1997; Pliszka, 1998).

Although several hypotheses have tried to explain this significant overlap of deficits, the precise underlying mechanisms are still unclear. It is assumed that the various hypotheses regarding these complex interrelationships are not mutually exclusive and that a number of causes may be acting in concert (Gillberg, 2003).

Regardless of the cause, the issue of co-existing deficits has important implications for the diagnosis, evaluation, treatment and prognosis of children with ADHD.

The disorders co-existing with ADHD have generally been divided into two groups (Adesman, 2003): psychiatric comorbidity (the most common disorders being oppositional-defiant and conduct disorder, anxiety disorder and depression) (Conner, Edward, Fletcher, Baird, Barkley, and Steingard 2003; Fischer, Barkley, Smallish, and Fletcher, 2002; Giedd, 2000; Pierce, 2003), and co-occurring neuro-developmental deficits in various domains. Predominant among these are deficits in motor (Fliers, Rommelse, Vermeulen, et al., 2008), language (Barbro, Thermlund, and Nettelbladt, 2006; Wassenberg, Hendriksen, Hurks., et al., 2010), cognitive (Frazier, Demarre, and Youngstrom, 2004) and sensory functioning.

Pertaining to the sensory domain, children with ADHD are frequently affected by deficiencies in sensory processing in general (Pfeiffer, Daly, Nicholls, and Gullo, 2014), and sensory modulation disorder in particular (Dunn and Bennett, 2002;; Mangeot, Miller, McIntosh, McGrath- Clarke, Simon, Hagerman., et al., 2001; Miller, Reisman, McIntosh, and Simon, 2001; Parush, Sohmer, Steinberg, and Kaitz, 1997; Yochman, Ornoy, and Parush, 2006).

SENSORY MODULATION DISORDER

Sensory processing is an encompassing term referring to the way that the nervous system manages incoming sensory information, including the reception, modulation, integration, perception and organization of sensory stimuli (Miller and Lane, 2000). The term *sensory modulation* relates to one specific component of this process and references both physiological reactions and behavioral responses (Miller et al., 2001). Physiologically, the term refers to the cellular mechanisms of habituation and excitation that alter the structure and/or function of nerve cells, affecting synaptic transmission (Kandel, 1991). This is a vital function, enabling the individual to focus on the most relevant environmental events that in any given situation support function and performance (Reeves, 2001).

Behaviorally, the term refers to the ability of an individual to regulate and organize the degree, intensity, and nature of responses to sensory input in a graded and adaptive manner (Lane, Miller, and Hanft, 2000).

Overall, one's ability to effectively modulate sensory input and respond in an adaptive manner has far-reaching effects on the individual's ability to engage in daily activities and quality of life (Dunn, 2001; Lane, 2002).

Individuals differ in their response to sensation with respect to the type, intensity and affective tone displayed, as well as to the onset and offset of the response (Ben-Sasson, Carter, and Briggs-Gowan, 2009). These differences influence peoples' interest in, tolerance for, and pleasure derived from sensations, which in turn affect their behavior and life choices (Dunn, 2001).

Thus, for example, some of us like to touch and be touched, while others prefer that people keep their distance; some are picky eaters and others are not; some have to jog intensely or need high volume music in order to remain calm, whereas others feel overwhelmed by the very same sensory experiences (Dunn, 2008). Individual differences such as these are normal and do not necessarily have a significant influence on overall daily life.

However, people with sensory modulation disorder experience more pervasive and clinically significant difficulties in modulating sensory input, to an extent that interferes with their participation in daily occupations and activities.

Sensory Modulation Disorder (SMD) is one subtype within the diagnosis of Sensory Processing Disorder. Sensory Processing Disorder (SPD) is a heterogeneous dysfunction that affects the manner in which individuals process and use sensory information for self-regulation, motor performance and function. Initially coined by Ayres (1972) as "sensory integration dysfunction", SPD is currently the diagnostic term most commonly used.

Three primary patterns of the disorder have been proposed: sensory discrimination disorder, sensory-based motor disorder and sensory modulation disorder (SMD) (Miller, Anzalone, Lane, Cermak, and Osten, 2007). This chapter focuses on SMD.

SMD is a recognized disorder in the Diagnostic Manual of the Interdisciplinary Council on Developmental and Learning Disorders (ICDL–DMIC, 2005) and the Zero to Three Diagnostic Classification of Mental Health and Developmental Disorders of Infancy and Early Childhood: Revised edition (DC: 0-3R) (Zero to Three, 2005). Even though certain symptoms of SMD are unique, this dysfunction has not yet been included as a separate disorder in the DSM or in the International Classification of Diseases (ICD) systems (Koziol and Budding, 2012). Nevertheless, the latest version of the DSM- 5 (APA, 2013) has included symptoms of hyper-or hypo-reactivity to sensory input as part of the diagnostic criteria of autism spectrum disorder (ASD), due to the fact that a high percentage of children with ASD present with sensory modulation disorder (Ben-Sasson, Hen, Fluss, Cermak, Engel- Yeger, and Gal 2009).

SMD refers to an individual's difficulty in responding to sensory stimuli with behavior that is graded and adaptive relative to the degree, nature, or intensity of the sensory information (Miller et al., 2007).

Three subtypes of SMD have been reported: sensory over-responsivity (SOR), sensory under-responsivity (SUR), and sensory seeking/craving (SS/C).

These subtypes can occur individually, or the disorder may manifest as a combination of symptoms from the three subtypes. The specific symptoms may involve only one or multiple sensory systems (e.g., tactile, vestibular, proprioceptive, visual, auditory, olfactory, and/or gustatory) (Dunn, 1997; Miller et al., 2007).

Children with *Sensory Over-Responsivity (SOR)* experience sensations more intensely and for longer durations than typically developing children. These children experience otherwise benign sensations as unpleasant, distracting or even painful, and respond with exaggerated avoidant and defensive behaviors that are inappropriate to the environmental demands. More intense responses are particularly evident in new situations, during transition periods and when the stimulus emerges unexpectedly. In addition, sensory input often has a summative effect. Thus, a sudden exaggerated response may occur to a seemingly trivial event as a result of the accumulation of antecedent sensory stimuli (Miller et al., 2007).

As previously mentioned, children with SOR may demonstrate over-responsivity to all types of sensory stimuli. Behavioral responses may commonly include avoidance of certain textures of clothing, aversive responses to touch or daily living tasks (e.g., showering, cutting fingernails or face washing), avoidance of everyday movement experiences (e.g., playing on playground equipment and sports activities), or over-responsivity to every-day smells (e.g., cleaning materials, shampoo, soap, perfumes), routine sounds (home appliances, people talking, doorbell ringing) and a reluctance to participate in social events (e.g., going to restaurants, attending parties, etc.).

Behaviors of children with SOR range from active, negative, impulsive, or aggressive responses such as temper tantrums, screaming and hostile behaviors, to more passive behaviors such as withdrawal or avoidance of the stimuli in order to ward off any additional exposure (Dunn, 2008; Miller, 2006). SOR has been identified as the most common type of SMD, reported to be found among approximately 80% of children referred for SMD (Schaaf, 2001).

In contrast, *Sensory Under-Responsivity (SUR)* is thought to result from nervous system hyposensitivity to sensory input. Children with SUR respond less to or take longer to respond to input. Under-responsivity may occur in only one or in multiple sensory systems.

Characteristic behaviors may, for example, manifest as a delayed or decreased response to extreme temperature or pain, a failure to be aware of people or objects in their environment, noxious smells and/or hearing one's name being called.

This lack of initial awareness to sensation may lead to withdrawn, self-absorbed and passive behavior, and a seeming lack of interest and motivation to initiate socialization and exploration. Children with SUR have difficulty listening, following directions, knowing where their body is in space and initiating movement. In order to become involved in a task or interaction, children with SUR need high-intensity, salient input (ICDL, 2005; Miller et al., 2007; Zero to three, 2005).

*Sensory Seeking /Craving (*SS/C*)*, another variant of SMD, describes children who seek out high intensity or increased durations of sensory stimulation and have an almost insatiable desire for sensory input. They engage energetically in actions that provide intense sensations in many varied modalities. Thus they tend to be constantly 'on the move', touching and/or crashing into people or objects, they may fixate on visually stimulating objects, seek loud sounds or unusual olfactory or gustatory experiences such as licking or chewing on things that are not edible or smelling objects. Difficulty in inhibiting such behaviors often leads to a disregard for others, as well as acting in a manner that is inappropriate and incompatible with a given environmental setting, such as continually moving and jumping in a setting that requires sedentary behavior (Dunn, 2000; Miller et al., 2007).

Since such sensory-seeking behaviors are often present in children exhibiting both over- and under-responsivity, some researchers have suggested that this subtype may be more reflective of a compensatory behavioral pattern undertaken to counteract the over or under-responsiveness of these children's nervous system, rather than a stand-alone SMD subtype (Reynolds and Lane, 2008).

The primary deficits resulting from all three subtypes of SMD are the individual's difficulty in grading or regulating responses to sensory stimuli and maintaining an optimal level of arousal (Kinnealey, Oliver, and Wilbarger, 1995; McIntosh, Miller, Shyu, and Hagerman 1999; Parham and Mailloux, 1996). In turn, these characteristics influence a person's attention, cognitive processing and emotional stability (Dunn, 1997; Lane, 2002; Parham and Mailloux, 1996). Possible attentional/cognitive manifestations of poor sensory modulation include distractibility, impulsiveness, disorganization and hyperactivity (Ayres, 1972; Cohn, Miller, and Tickle-Degnen, 2000, Miller et al., 2001). The affective manifestations may include anxiety, depression, anger, hostility, emotional lability and poor self-regulation (Cohn et al., 2000; Miller et al., 2001).

A diagnosis of SMD is made only when the resulting behaviors significantly affect a child's daily life. Children with SMD have been reported to have problems with functional performance in all areas of daily living such as dressing, meal and bath times, play, and social interactions (Bar-Shalita, Vatine, and Parush, 2008). Moreover, this disorder can profoundly and negatively impact the child's and his/her family's quality of life, ability to engage in and enjoy social interactions and participation in daily routines (Bar-Shalita et al. 2008; Brett-Green, Miller, Schoen, and Nielsen, 2010). Evidence indicates that manifestations of SMD during childhood/adolescence continue into adulthood (Brown, Tollefson, Dunn, Cromwell, and Filion, 2001).

Empirical research supporting SMD as an independent clinical condition is still limited, although accumulating evidence indicates unique behavioral and physiological characteristics of children with SMD that are different from those of typically developing children.

Most of the research on the physiological manifestations of SMD has been conducted on children with SOR. Current research on the underlying neurobiology of SMD is based on the hypothesis that autonomic and central nervous system processes are affected (Miller et al., 2012).

The research relating to autonomic nervous system function in children with SMD originated with the pioneering work of Dr. A. Jean Ayres, an occupational therapist and neuroscientist. This conceptualization is supported by current clinical observations that many children with SMD-SOR exhibit 'fight or flight' and defensive responses to one or more types of sensory stimuli which are not perceived as overwhelming by typically developing children (Ayres, 1964; Brett-Green et al., 2010).

Research indicates that children with SMD were shown to have greater frequency and higher magnitude electrodermal responses (EDR- a measure of sympathetic nervous system activity) to sensory stimuli than typically developing children. In addition, children with SMD were shown to habituate more slowly following repeated stimulation (McIntosh et al., 1999). The results of another study by Schaaf, Miller, Seawell, and O'Keefe (2003) revealed that a sample of children with disturbances in sensory modulation had statistically significant lower cardiac vagal tone and a lower heart period than those in the control group which comprised typically developing children, suggesting that they have less effective parasympathetic functioning.

The sympathetic and parasympathetic responses found in these studies were hypothesized as contributing to the inability of children with SMD-SOR to moderate the degree, intensity, and type of response to typical environmental sensory stimuli.

In the area of central nervous system research, studies set out to examine potential brain processes underlying SMD. Primary evidence that children with SMD display different brain processing mechanisms compared to children who are typically developing, was presented in an auditory event-related potential study (Davies and Gavin, 2007; Davies, Chang, and Gavin, 2009) using electroencephalographic (EEG) measures. In these studies, children with SMD did not exhibit the expected increase in response following increased intense stimulation. These findings may be indicative of less organized brain processing to simple auditory stimuli. Children with SMD had more difficulty filtering out repeated or irrelevant sensory information and did not show an improvement with age, as did typically developing children in sensory gating (a measure of the CNS's ability to inhibit responses to redundant or irrelevant sensory stimuli).

Studying simultaneous multisensory auditory and somatosensory input in children with SMD-SOR, Brett-Green and colleagues (2010) found that during both early and later stages of sensory information processing, multisensory integration (MSI) was detected mainly over the fronto-central regions of the cortex, whereas in typically developing children (Brett-Green, Miller, Gavin, and Davis, 2008) MSI was observed in the ipsilateral cortex and in midline cortical regions. Furthermore, children with SMD-SOR showed smaller amplitude MSI responses in midline and frontal cortical regions, and showed an absence of ipsilateral integration. The researchers concluded that the automatic integration of multisensory stimuli that generally occurs in lower level cortical regions early in the course of sensory information processing may not occur in children with SMD-SOR. Instead, higher-level frontal MSI processes may be engaged. The possible ramification of this finding may explain why children with SMD-SOR tend to attend to all environmental stimuli, meaningful or not.

Bar-Shalita, Vatine, Seltzer, and Parush (2009) tested somatosensory thresholds and suprathresholds using quantitative sensory methods. Their research provided preliminary evidence indicating that children with SMD were not different than their typical peers in threshold detection (with the exception of cool detection), but perceived higher and more lasting pain intensity to suprathreshold pinprick and to prickly stimuli. This finding highlights the increased sensitivity of such children to painful stimuli and, possibly, central nervous system involvement.

A recent investigation of the white matter in the brains of children with SPD via MR imaging demonstrated a specific reduction of the white matter microstructure, primarily in the posterior cerebral tracts. Moreover, the reduced posterior white matter microstructural integrity correlated directly with the atypical sensory behavior of these children (Owen, Marco, Desai, Fourie, Harris, Hill, et al., 2013).

Overall, these studies, suggest the existence of a biological basis for sensory processing dysfunctions such as SMD, implicating affected autonomic nervous system and involvement of primary sensory cortical areas, higher-order multi-sensory integration cortical regions as well as abnormal CNS microstructure.

It is important to note that in addition, external contextual factors have also been shown to play a vital role in mediating responsivity in SMD. The Ecological Model of Sensory Modulation (Miller, et al., 2001) highlights the importance of understanding the effects of external ecological factors (culture, environment, relationships and tasks) on the functioning of individuals with SMD. The developers of this model propose that SMD results from the dynamic interaction between the individual's *internal* sensory, attentional and emotional capacities and these *external* factors. Accordingly, they state that a "just right match" between internal and external dimensions will result in adaptive functional performance.

COMORBIDITY: ADHD AND SMD

Differential diagnosis between ADHD and SMD is often challenging, since these disorders share several clinical characteristics For example, in the face of adverse sensory stimulation, and given their inherent difficulty in screening out irrelevant stimuli, the behavioral responses of children with sensory over-responsivity (SOR) may manifest as impaired attention, distractibility, impulsivity, hyperactivity, or some combination of these; all of which also represent the core symptoms of ADHD (Miller, Nielsen, and Schoen, 2012; Lane, Reynolds, and Thacker, 2010; Yochman, Alon- Beery, Sribman, and Parush, 2013).

Although this symptom overlap has been documented primarily with regard to SOR, researchers have noted that symptoms of ADHD may overlap with other subtypes of SMD as well (Miller et al., 2012). Thus, children characterized as sensory seeking/craving (SS/C) may show poor impulse control, inattention, inappropriate movement and disorganization; behaviors which are similar to the hyperactivity- impulsivity subtype of ADHD. Likewise, children with sensory under-responsivity (SUR) often present with attention difficulties, such as being unaware when spoken to or inattentive when asked to follow directions. In some aspects, this behavior resembles the inattention subtype of ADHD (Miller, 2006; Miller et al., 2012).

In addition to their shared behavioural characteristics, differential diagnosis between ADHD and SMD is further complicated by a high prevalence of comorbidity, such as has been revealed in several studies.

In view of the high comorbidity and overlap of symptoms, an increasing amount of research in recent years has focused on obtaining a better understanding of the relationship between these disorders. Empirical evidence is vital in order to clearly distinguish between ADHD and SMD and further clarify their etiologies. Refining and improving the diagnostic accuracy within and between these diagnoses will in turn support the development of appropriate, optimal interventions.

The following section will provide a review of the research on the relationship between ADHD and SMD, followed by a discussion of the theoretical and clinical implications.

Studies relating to this issue can broadly be divided into three main categories:

a) the prevalence of SMD/ADHD and their co-existence, b) the sensory profiles of children with ADHD, and c) the differentiation between SMD and ADHD.

PREVALENCE OF ADHD/SMD

Many studies have reported the prevalence of ADHD among population-based samples of preschool and school aged children (Feldman and Reiff, 2014; Froehlich, Lanphear, Epstein, Barbaresi, Katusic, and Kahn, 2007). The recent DSM-5 (APA, 2013) criteria report a prevalence rate of 5% in most cultures, although several researchers argue that the true rates are much higher (Barbaresi, Katusic, Colligan, Pankratz, Weaver, and Weber, 2002; Robison, Sclar, Skaer and Galin, 2004).

By contrast, few studies have attempted to document the prevalence of SMD in the general pediatric population. Results of these studies indicate that its prevalence is similar to that of ADHD, with estimated rates of 5-16 % (Ahn, Miller, Milberger, and Mcintosh, 2004; Ben-Sasson et al., 2009; Gouze, Hopkins, Lebailly, and Lavigne, 2009).

While prevalence studies have been conducted for each clinical population separately, to date, no wide scale study has been done with the specific aim of documenting the prevalence of co-occurring ADHD and SMD among either clinical or population-based samples. Nevertheless, several studies relating to various other research questions regarding the relationship between ADHD and SMD have reported the percentage of co-occurrence of ADHD and SMD within their study samples. In general, these results indicate that compared to the prevalence rates of SMD among typically developing children, the percentage of SMD among defined populations of children with ADHD is much higher. In fact, some studies have indicated that as many as half the children with ADHD will also exhibit SMD.

Thus, for example, Lane and colleagues (2010) performed a study on the relationship between anxiety, SMD and ADHD. Within the 84 children aged 6-12 years old included in their study, 39 were diagnosed as ADHD and of these children, 46% also had SOR. An even larger percentage of coexistence was reported by Parush et al. (2007) in a study examining somatosensory functioning deficits among 5-11 year-old boys with ADHD; 69% of the 67 boys with ADHD who participated in the study were found to be tactilely over-responsive. Similar findings were also found among younger preschool children with ADHD. For instance, in a study that set out to develop a comprehensive profile of the sensory, motor, language and intellectual functioning of non-referred preschool children with ADHD in comparison to typically developing children, 46% of the 49 children in the ADHD group had co-occurring SMD, whereas only 9% of the 48 typically developing children had SMD (Yochman, Ornoy, and Parush, 2006).

Similarly, various other studies have also reported a substantial proportion of children with ADHD together with co-occurring SMD (i.e Mangeot et al., 2001; Miller et al., 2012; Reynolds, Lane, and Gennings, 2009).

Additional data on the co-occurrence of these two disorders was obtained from a study conducted to standardize the Leiter International Performance Scale Revised IQ test (Roid and Miller, 1997). As part of the standardization process, a nationally stratified sample of 2,410 typically developing children were screened for both the attentional symptoms of ADHD and the sensory symptoms of SMD. From the total sample, 7.5 % had symptoms of either sensory or attention impairments or both. Of the children with reported symptoms, 32% had symptoms of only ADHD, 28% had symptoms of only SMD, and 40% were reported to have symptoms of both disorders (Miller, 2006).

In summary, the mounting evidence from studies indicates that the comorbidity of ADHD and SMD is not a marginal phenomenon. Moreover, given that these findings were evident in studies that examined both clinical as well as community-based samples, it cannot be argued that they were skewed as a result of referral or selection bias. Nevertheless, it is important to emphasize that these studies also included children who had only sensory or only attentional impairment, lending support to the claim that they are separate disorders.

SENSORY PROFILES OF CHILDREN WITH ADHD

Studies in this area of research investigated the characteristic sensory processing profile of children with ADHD compared to typical children using both behavioral and physiological measures.

Comparison between Children with ADHD and Typically Developing Children on Sensory Behavioral Measures

The behavioral measures used in these studies consisted mainly of caregiver questionnaires aimed at providing a detailed description of how children respond to sensory events in daily life. Although parents' reports are subjective by nature, parents are also the most likely source for obtaining a rich and detailed picture of a young child's responses to sensory events across time. In addition, behaviors related to a child's responses to aversive sensory stimuli in daily life situations are often difficult to observe directly in a controlled or time-restrained situation (Ben-Sasson et al., 2009; De Los Reyes and Kazdin, 2005).

Among the most commonly used standardized sensory-behavioral questionnaires are the Sensory Profile Questionnaire (SP; Dunn, 1999) and the Short Sensory Profile (SSP; McIntosh, Miller, and Dunn, 1999a). The SP questionnaire aims to identify sensory processing deficits. It comprises 125 items related to the assessment of sensory modulation (i.e., the ability to grade the degree, intensity and nature of responses to sensory input), as well as to the behavioral and emotional responses resulting from sensory modulation deficits.

Scoring involves a 5-point Likert scale corresponding to the frequency of each behavior (i.e., 1=always, 5=never). Several scores can be obtained, including scores on 14 Sensory Profile sub-sections (inter alia, processing in all individual sensory systems), four basic patterns of sensory processing- seeking, avoiding, sensitivity, and registration (each of which reflects a combination of a person's unique neurological threshold and self-regulation strategy), and nine Sensory Profile factors (reflecting the child's level of responsivity , i.e., over and under responsiveness to sensory input across sensory systems). The reliability and validity of this evaluation has been established and it has been shown to significantly discriminate between children with and without SMD (Dunn, 1999; Erner and Dunn, 1998).

The Short Sensory Profile (SSP; McIntosh et al., 1999), also a reliable and valid standardized caregiver questionnaire, consists of 38 behavioral statements originating from the longer Sensory Profile. This questionnaire was designed to be a screening tool, having the advantage of being short and therefore useful for research. It thus provides a somewhat less comprehensive and detailed description of sensory processing than the SP. The individual items are arranged into seven categories: *tactile sensitivity, taste/smell sensitivity, under-responsive/seeks sensation, auditory filtering, visual/auditory sensitivity, low energy /weak, and movement sensitivity.*

Using these tools, several studies have described the sensory processing abilities of children with ADHD. In 2001, Mangeot and colleagues compared sensory processing patterns between 26 children with ADHD and 30 typically developing children (ages 5-13) on various measures, including the SSP. The results of the SSP showed significantly lower scores in six of the seven subscales among children with ADHD, particularly in seeks sensation and auditory filtering, as well as sensitivity to tactile, auditory/ visual, taste/smell stimuli.

Miller et al. (2012) also utilizing the SSP, also revealed that children referred for ADHD had significantly poorer scores compared to typically developing children on seeks sensation, auditory filtering, tactile, auditory/visual sensitivity, and low energy/weak. No differences were found on taste/smell and movement sensitivity.

A more in-depth and detailed description of the sensory processing abilities of children with ADHD was obtained in studies that utilized the full Sensory Profile. For instance, Dunn and Bennett (2002) compared parents' perceptions of sensory behaviors of 70 children with ADHD aged 3 to 15, selected from treatment centers, to those of a matched group of 70 typically developing children. Results indicated that the sensory responsiveness of children with ADHD differed significantly from that of children without ADHD on all 14 sub-sections of the Sensory Profile. The majority of items in which the most significant differences were observed were clustered into four factors: sensory seeking, emotionally reactive, inattention /distractibility, and fine motor.

Similar findings were obtained in studies from other countries. In a Sensory Profile study performed on Israeli preschool children with ADHD, Yochman and colleagues (2004) compared the functioning of 48 children with ADHD from a community sample with a matched group of 46 typically developing children. The results were compelling, revealing that even among a non- referred population, children with ADHD scored significantly worse in 11 out of the 14 section scores, and in 6 out of 9 factor scores. Likewise, using the Sensory Profile, Cheung and Siu (2009), verified greater impairments in sensory processing in Chinese children with ADHD compared to children without ADHD.

Overall, these findings seem to support the view that across a number of sensory modalities, children with ADHD exhibit significantly more difficulties in sensory processing than typically developing children

When relating to these results, several issues must be taken into account.

Behavioral measures, such as the SP questionnaire, include items which address not only sensory modulation but also behaviors considered to be derivatives of sensory modulation dysfunction, such as inattention and social-emotional functioning. Moreover, two sections of the SSP, specifically the subtests relating to *seeks sensation* and *auditory filtering*, overlap with items describing ADHD in the DSM (Miller et al., 2012). Therefore, in order to truly examine sensory modulation in children with ADHD, it is important to try and extract those behaviors that relate specifically to sensory modulation, as opposed to those that could also reflect either the core symptoms of ADHD (such as inattention), or behaviors that are not innate but are nevertheless characteristic of the ADHD population (such as social-emotional difficulties) (Wehmeier, Schacht, and Barkley, 2010).

Nevertheless, a careful analysis of the results of the above studies indicates that children with ADHD do indeed perform significantly worse on items that represent sensory modulation issues per se. For example, children with ADHD are more sensitive to touch, vestibular and oral sensory stimuli (Dunn and Bennett, 2002; Yochman et al., 2004). Thus, behavioral measures seem to indicate that when compared to typical children, children with ADHD are at increased risk of deficits in sensory modulation abilities, over and above the core symptoms of ADHD.

In addition, it is important to take into account that despite the evidence showing that children with ADHD have noticeable difficulties in sensory processing, a certain percentage of the children in these studies displayed typical sensory processing. This variability emphasizes the importance of relating to the individual child and not only to the characteristics of the group.

Comparison between Children with ADHD and Typically Developing Children on Physiological Measures

A number of studies have examined the response to sensory stimuli of children with ADHD in comparison to typically developing children by measuring objective physiological markers. These studies have revealed the presence of significantly different patterns of sensory processing and modulation. One of the more frequently used measures in these studies is electro-dermal reactivity (EDR), a measure of sympathetic nervous system activity. The EDR records changes in electrical conductance of the skin associated with eccrine sweat gland activity, in reaction to novel, startling or threatening stimuli and during both positive and negative emotional events (McIntosh, Miller, Shyu, and Hagerman, 1999b; Miller et al., 2001). A number of studies have investigated EDR reactivity patterns among children with ADHD in an attempt to further refine our knowledge about this population and to describe their characteristic sensory profiles This methodology was employed since previous studies have shown that the reactivity of children with SMD showed greater frequency and magnitude of electrodermal responses to sensory stimulation, and a slower habituation rate following repeated stimulation in comparison to typically developing children (McIntosh et al., 1999b; Miller et al., 2001).

The findings regarding possible differences in EDR reactivity between children with and without ADHD were inconsistent. In 2001, Mangeot et al. compared the EDRs of children with ADHD to typically developing children. The sensory challenge protocol included the presentation of sensory stimuli in various sensory domains (olfactory, auditory, visual, tactile and vestibular). Findings demonstrated that in comparison to the children in the control group, children in the ADHD group displayed a larger initial reaction to the presentation of the stimulus in each domain, followed by a faster than normal habituation to repeated stimulation. In contrast, using the same sensory protocol, Miller et al. (2012) found no significant differences in the magnitude of EDR between children with ADHD and typically developing children in all sensory domains. The researchers concluded that a lack of consensus remains as to whether the physiological reactivity of children with ADHD is smaller, larger or the same as in typically developing children. The inconsistency of research findings may be due to methodological variability between studies. Another possible explanation is that children with ADHD do not represent a homogenous group, and thus their patterns of autonomic nervous system arousal may differ according to subgroups within ADHD (Mangeot et al., 2001; Miller et al., 2012).

In summary, although comparing the characteristics of sensory processing among children with and without ADHD requires a more sophisticated level of analysis than behavioral studies alone can provide, very few studies have incorporated objective physiological measures into their research. The sparse evidence appears to indicate that some aspects of sensory processing among children with ADHD differ from typically developing children. The limited data, coupled with the fact that empirical research on the physiological manifestations of SMD is a fairly new and insufficiently examined area of study, makes it difficult to draw clear conclusions.

DIFFERENTIATING SMD FROM ADHD

As discussed above, many children with ADHD have sensory processing difficulties characteristic of SMD. Nevertheless, the basic assumption of the majority of researchers is that SMD is a separate condition frequently co-occurring with other disorders, including ADHD. In order to be considered a separate disorder, SMD must have documented convergent and discriminant validity, demonstrating that the characteristics of a group found to have SMD occur reliably and that this exact pattern of symptoms is not replicated in any other diagnostic group (Miller et al., 2001).

Accumulating research, albeit limited, has been aimed at confirming that SMD is indeed a valid dysfunction, distinct from other recognized disorders. The field of research regarding comorbidity versus differentiation of SMD from other disorders addresses a variety of diagnostic groups, such as ASD (Ben- Sasson et al., 2009), Fragile X (Baranek, David, and Poe, 2006), OCD (Hazen et al., 2008) and anxiety disorders (Hofmann and Bitran, 2007).

The present review, however, addresses only the research differentiating SMD from ADHD.

To address this issue, several studies have compared children with a sole diagnosis of ADHD to children with a sole diagnosis of SMD in an attempt to describe the unique profile of each population.

The main emphasis in these studies was to compare these two groups in relation to the core symptoms of both SMD and ADHD in order to distinguish characteristics that might discriminate and/or overlap in the two conditions.

Some studies have also compared children with these disorders on measures of social-emotional functioning. Difficulties in this domain are associated with both SMD and ADHD and could, therefore, possibly contribute to the behavioral similarity of these disorders.

The following section will briefly summarize these studies. Some of the studies described also included a comparison between children diagnosed with either SMD or ADHD to typically developing children (see previous section) as well as to children with a dual diagnosis.

However, this discussion will focus primarily on results that relate to characteristics distinguishing between children with SMD and those with ADHD, thus lending support to the contention that they are separate disorders.

Ognibene (2002) was among the first to address the hypothesis that children with ADHD and SMD would exhibit opposing profiles on two characteristic manifestations of each individual disorder. Specifically, it was expected that children with SMD–SOR would demonstrate slow habituation to repeated sensation, but no difficulty in response inhibition - a common characteristic of children with ADHD (Brown, 2013). Conversely, it was assumed that ADHD symptoms would be associated with poor response inhibition, but would not relate to sensory habituation. As expected, results indicated that children with SMD and those with ADHD demonstrated opposing profiles in most, but not all cases.

Miller et al. (2012) compared behaviors and physiological reactions of 70 children with SMD, 37 with ADHD, 12 with a dual diagnosis of SMD and ADHD and 57 typically developing children. The researchers examined various characteristics, employing several measures of sensation, attention and emotion. In the specific comparison between children with SMD and ADHD, significant differences on several of these measures were revealed.

Results relating to sensory processing showed that on the SSP parental report, children with SMD had significantly poorer scores on the majority of subtests (tactile sensitivity, taste/smell sensitivity, visual/auditory sensitivity, movement sensitivity and low energy/ weak), mostly within the clinically impaired range. No differences were found on the subtests of seeks sensation and auditory filtering, two sections of the SSP that include items which are also characteristic of children with ADHD.

Moreover, children with SMD exhibited greater electro-dermal reactivity magnitudes to auditory, visual, and movement stimuli, although no group differences were found in the olfactory and tactile domains.

Thus, the results of the sensory measures indicated that although various studies have shown that children with ADHD display sensory problems in comparison to typically developing children, when compared to children with SMD, results revealed a different and significantly more impaired sensory profile among the children with SMD versus ADHD.

Results relating to ADHD symptomatology, as measured by the SNAP-IV- a norm referenced parent scale (Swanson, 1992), showed that children with ADHD had significantly worse scores than children with SMD on the inattention subtest. However, the hyperactivity/ impulsivity subtest failed to differentiate between the groups. These results indicate that while differences exist, there is nevertheless some overlap with respect to ADHD symptomatology.

Emotional functioning was assessed by the Child Behavior Checklist (CBCL; Achenbach, 1991) and the Leiter International Performance Scale-revised (Roid and Miller, 1997). The findings indicated that children with SMD had more somatic complaints, were more likely to be withdrawn or anxious/depressed, and had more difficulty adapting and being flexible in the presence of unexpected occurrences. Although these findings support the hypothesis that children with sensory difficulties are particularly vulnerable to emotional problems as a result of experiencing their sensory environment as unpredictable and overwhelming (Miller et al., 2001; Miller et al., 2012), it should be noted that the scores of children with SMD were within the normal ranges.

Lane, Reynolds, and Thacker (2010) attempted to differentiate between groups of children with ADHD, SMD (specifically SOR), a dual diagnosis of ADHD and SOR and typically developing children based on neuroendocrine levels (salivary cortisol), EDR reactivity and behaviors reflecting anxiety. A change in salivary cortisol levels is considered to be a physiological reflection of a stress response (Hanrahan, McCarthy, Kleiber, Lutgendorf, and Tsalikian, 2006). The children's cortisol levels were measured prior to and following the presentation of sensory stimuli. Cortisol levels had been shown to differentiate between children with SMD and typically developing children in previous studies (Reynolds et al., 2009). A measure of anxiety (Revised Children's Manifest Anxiety Scale - RCMAS), was included in this study, since previous studies had documented a link between anxiety and both ADHD (Schatz and Rostain, 2006) and SMD (Ben- Sasson et al., 2007; Hofmann and Bitran, 2007).

The findings did not find statistical differences between children with SOR and children with ADHD in levels of neuroendocrine stress and electrodermal markers. In contrast, significant group differences were found on the anxiety measure. Children with a dual diagnosis of ADHD and SOR differed significantly from children with ADHD on the physio-logic anxiety subscale, and from children with SOR alone on all three subscales: physiologic anxiety, worry/over-sensitivity and social concern/concentration.

These results suggest that although some aspects of anxiety may characterize ADHD in general, other aspects may be more specifically tied to SOR. In addition, the finding that children with both ADHD and SOR are more likely to show higher anxiety levels than children with only one diagnosis emphasizes the importance of relating to this specific sub-group when attempting to differentiate between SMD and ADHD.

Yet another study which contributed to this body of knowledge is a study performed by Parush et al. (2007) who examined children's tactile sensory processing by measuring somato-sensory evoked potentials (SEP). SEP is the averaged response of the peripheral and central components of the somatosensory pathway, reflecting the transmission of neural signals along the dorsal column medial lemeniscus pathway between peripheral neurons and the cortex.

Their study population comprised children with ADHD divided into two sub groups: children with ADHD only and children with ADHD and SMD, focusing specifically on children who exhibit tactile over- responsivity. Comparison between these groups demonstra-ted significantly larger than normal amplitudes of central components for children with a dual diagnosis of ADHD and tactile over-responsivity. No group differences were found on the amplitude of the peripheral component of the SEP.

These results provide evidence of a link between sensory over-responsivity and atypical central neural processing that is more likely associated with tactile over-responsivity or a combination of tactile over-responsivity and ADHD, than to ADHD per se.

A recently published study (Yochman et al., 2013) compared the profiles of children with SMD to those of children with ADHD with respect to attention and sensation, using measures applicable for clinical use.

Several sensory measures were included. The Fabric Prickliness Test (FPT) and the Von Frey Monofilament Test used in this study are based on quantitative sensory testing (QST), a psychophysical approach used to characterize somatosensory hypersensitivity in a non-invasive but rigorous manner (Arendt- Nielsen and Yarnitsky, 2009; Hansson et al., 2007; Verdugo and Ochoa, 1992).

Both tests have been shown to be valid methods of determining pain levels in children, as well as for distinguishing between children with and without SMD in their perception of pain and pain 'after sensation' (Bar-Shalita et al., 2009). The study also included the Evaluation of Sensory Processing Questionnaire (ESP; Parham and Johnson-Ecker, 2002), a care-giver questionnaire designed to identify behaviors indicative of sensory processing problems [The ESP is the predecessor of the Sensory Processing Measure Home questionnaire (SPM) (Kuhaneck et al., 2007)].

Results indicated significantly greater sensory difficulties among children in the SMD group on all sensory measures. Specifically, children with SMD reported higher scores as a response to punctate pain, as well as differences in the measures of pain 'after-sensation'. In other words, in children with SMD, the pain sensation lingered longer than in children with ADHD. In addition, the results of the parent questionnaire showed significantly lower scores in three of the six subtests (i.e., taste and smell, tactile and motion /vestibular).

Surprisingly, on the various attention components measured by the Test of Everyday Attention for Children (TEA-Ch; Manly et al., 1999), children with ADHD did not perform significantly worse than the children with SMD on any of the sub- tests (selective, sustained, divided and switched attention).

In addition to sensory and attention components, this study was the first to compare these two diagnostic populations in their unique expression of participation limitations across multiple areas of functioning. As participation is directly related to health and represents the highest level of functioning (WHO, 2001), this variable was investigated in an attempt to determine whether functional participation represented an additional important factor to consider in the differential diagnosis of these populations. However, no group differences were found in most areas of participation, suggesting that children's specific clinical diagnoses may not be a major factor in determining their participation profiles.

Others have addressed the question of SMD as an independent diagnostic entity by providing evidence that a subset of children with symptoms of SMD do not qualify for other diagnoses, including ADHD. For example, Van Hulle, Schmidt, and Goldsmith (2012) conducted a study aimed at investigating the distinctiveness of SOR utilizing a behavior-genetic framework within a large community-based sample of school-age twins and their families. They concluded that although SOR is a relatively frequent comorbid condition with recognized diagnoses, it was found to occur independently of common childhood psychiatric diagnoses (such as ADHD, CD, ODD, anxiety, phobia and depression) in nearly half of all children who screened positive for SOR. The authors' tentative conclusion was that some support exists for a subset of children with SMD who do not qualify for other diagnoses. Their findings lend support to Goldsmith, Van Hulle, Arneson, Schrieber, and Gernsbacher's (2006) population-based twin study in which it was reported that auditory and tactile SOR were largely distinct from other common childhood disorders.

DISCUSSION

A review of the literature reveals that co-occurring deficits in ADHD is one of the most frequently explored aspects of this disorder. Thus far, the research regarding the link between ADHD and SMD is still relatively limited (Ghanizadeh, 2011). It is vital for more studies to be performed on this topic to expand our current understanding of the relationship between ADHD and SMD. Such studies will undoubtedly have important implications for both theory and practice with regard to these disorders.

However, according to the research performed thus far, the accumulating evidence strongly suggests that sensory modulation difficulties should be considered when planning interventions for children with ADHD.

As discussed in this chapter, the literature has revealed that a relatively high percentage of children with ADHD have been found to have co-occurring SMD and present with significantly more atypical sensory related behaviors than typically developing children.

Nonetheless, while research indicates a link between ADHD and SMD, preliminary evidence also suggests dissociation between these disorders, denoting that SMD is a separate clinical condition which frequently co- occurs with ADHD.

Specifically, SMD has been found to exist in the absence of ADHD and vice versa. Furthermore, research has demonstrated that a unique profile exists for each individual diagnosis. Studies have thus consistently revealed a different and significantly more impaired sensory profile among children with SMD compared to children with ADHD. In addition, some studies have found significant differences between these populations on measures of ADHD symptomology and emotional functioning, although these domains have received very limited attention and results were less conclusive compared to the sensory domain.

These findings raise questions regarding the mutual interdependence of these deficits. This issue is further complicated in view of the limited research done regarding the etiology of SMD (Koziol and Budding, 2012).

The conclusion of some investigators who consider SMD and ADHD to be separate diagnostic categories (Miller et al., 2012) is congruent with the additive model of comorbidity (Angold et al., 1999; Gillberg et al., 2004). This model suggests that co-existing deficits reflect the presence of two distinct disorders that may co-occur in the same individual but are unlinked either etiologically or sequentially. However, studies have yet to provide a satisfactory explanation as to which underlying brain mechanisms generate these differences (Koziol and Budding, 2012).

Another possible argument is that ADHD and co-existing SMD do share a common etiology. For example, Lane et al., (2010) have suggested that SMD and ADHD may share certain underlying neurobiological mechanisms. They maintain that it is possible that both the responses of children with sensory over-responsivity to sensory stimuli they find bothersome, such as striking out or moving to avoid the offending input, as well as the hyperactive-impulsive symptoms of ADHD, may be related to 'bottom-up' processes that are stimulus driven. Nigg (2006) proposed that the mechanisms involved in these processes may be related to striatal or limbic activation.

An alternative explanation posits that specific combinations of co-existing disorders may in fact represent distinct subtypes within the ADHD spectrum, with different clinical presentations, etiology factors, course and responses to treatment. Accordingly, Lane and colleagues (2010) have raised the question as to whether SMD may serve as a moderating variable in the definition of ADHD subtypes (ADHD with and without SMD). Based on their findings, they propose that there may be a subgroup of children with ADHD that is different from other children with ADHD by the presence of sensory over- responsivity symptoms, either with or without anxiety.

This would have specific clinical implications, since behaviors stemming from different underlying central nervous system processes would call for different types of treatment. A case in point relates to the treatment of children with comorbid ADHD and anxiety. It is generally accepted that dopamine hypo-function plays a pivotal role in the neurobiology of ADHD, as is also evident from the beneficial effects of stimulant medications on ADHD symptoms (Nigg, 2005). Nevertheless, children with comorbid ADHD and anxiety tend to respond poorly to medication, which may result from a difference in the underlying central nervous system process. Thus, the link to catecholamine dysfunction may not be as clear in this subgroup (Levy, 2004).

When considering the various hypotheses regarding the relationship between SMD and ADHD, one must also take into account the possibility of a sequential relationship, in which one disorder creates an increased risk for symptoms of the other. Thus, in certain instances, a child presenting with a primary deficit in sensory modulation may have secondary behavioral symptoms of hyperactivity, impulsivity and inattention.

It is also important to note that the diagnostic process itself may partially contribute to the high estimates of comorbidity reported in some studies. Koziol and Budding (2012) remarked that a categorically behaviorally defined diagnostic system, such as that applied in diagnosing both ADHD and SMD, invites diagnostic overlap and ambiguity as a result of the common symptoms used to describe each of these disorders in the diagnostic rating scales.

Clearly, additional research is necessary to clarify the underlying processes of SMD as well as the precise nature of the relationship between SMD and ADHD. It seems that the heterogeneity of impairments experienced by these children cannot adequately be explained by any one underlying cause, nor does it follow that the various hypotheses are mutually exclusive.

In addition to the theoretical implications, the existence of co-existing deficits among children with SMD and ADHD is of important clinical significance. In considering the high rate of various comorbid impairments found among children with ADHD, the American Academy of Pediatrics recommended that children referred due to behavioral symptoms suggestive of ADHD be routinely and systematically screened for other comorbid disorders (Adesman, 2003). Thus, it seems apt that co-occurring sensory modulation dysfunction should be considered in the diagnostic process of children referred for suspected ADHD.

This presents a diagnostic challenge for clinicians resulting from the overlap in symptoms found in both these disorders, as the data derived from assessment tools used to diagnose SMD (i.e., standardized questionnaires, clinical assessment and interviews), would also reflect the presence of some symptoms of ADHD. Thus, further effort needs to be invested to develop tools which can reliably distinguish between ADHD and SMD. That is, measures are needed that can help determine whether a primary sensory deficit underlies the child's behavioral symptoms, or whether the child presents with co-occurring deficits. These measures would need to demonstrate a higher level of specificity than those used to differentiate between SMD and typically developing children alone.

There is another important advantage in pursuing the identification of SMD in a child suspected of having ADHD, especially among preschool children. The diagnosis of ADHD in preschoolers is complicated by the fact that some of the symptomatic behaviors of ADHD are considered typical and age-related among young preschool children (Byrne et al., 2001; Sonuga - Barke et al., 2005). However, in general, children with SMD can be identified at an earlier age than children with ADHD since symptoms considered diagnostic of SMD are frequently apparent before the emergence of the core symptoms of ADHD (Miller et al., 2012). Thus, presenting symptoms of an additional neurological dysfunction, such as SMD, in a preschool child should alert the clinician to the possibility of comorbid ADHD.

With respect to the intervention process, treatment for children with ADHD should reflect a holistic approach that takes into account the multiple needs of the child, including potential problems in sensory modulation. Studies have demonstrated that co-occurring difficulties increase the risk of long-term difficulties, as opposed to children with isolated problems who are more likely to show a better outcome (Gillberg and Kadesjo, 2000).

It seems, therefore, that failure to relate to coexisting SMD may lead to a sub-optimal treatment plan. Hence, when necessary, treatment should include approaches such as those provided by occupational therapists, which target the specific sensory modulation deficits of the child in order to increase participation in activities in all of his/her primary environments, including at home, school, and in the community (Miller, Coll, and Schoen, 2007).

The theoretical and clinical implications derived from the literature need to take into account several issues which could influence our ability to arrive at more definitive conclusions.

Firstly, as mentioned previously, additional empirical evidence is required due to the paucity of research in this area. In addition, the methodological limitations of some of the existing studies may have adversely affected the findings. These limitations include, for example: small convenience samples, partially due to the difficulty of identifying participants with only one diagnosis; insufficient diagnostic criteria for each of the study groups; a large degree of variability within each diagnostic group due to lack of definition of specific sub-types of ADHD or SMD; insufficient controlling for the co- existence of SMD and ADHD in the study samples (e.g., lack of screening for ADHD in SMD participants).

Furthermore, different research methodology employed in the various studies complicates comparison between results, for example, variations in the inclusion criteria for study samples and in the assessment tools used to evaluate the constructs of sensation, attention and emotion. Despite these limitations, the research to date regarding the patterns of sensory modulation among children with ADHD undoubtedly broadens our ability to consider factors that might be influencing a child's behavior. This broader perspective can guide us towards providing the appropriate interventions which hopefully will improve the quality of life for these children.

REFERENCES

Achenbach, T. M. (1991). *Manual for the Child Behavior Checklist/4-18 and 1991 profile*. Burlington, VT: University of Vermont, Department of Psychiatry.

Adesman, A. (2003). A diagnosis of ADHD? Don't overlook the probability of comorbidity. *Contemporary Pediatrics*, 20, 91-112.

Ahn, R. R., Miller, L. J., Milberger, S., and McIntosh, D. N. (2004). Prevalence of parents' perceptions of sensory processing disorders among kindergarten children. *American Journal of Occupational Therapy*, 58, 287–302.

Angold, A., Costello, J. and Erkanli, A. (1999). Comorbidity. *Journal of Child Psychology and Psychiatry*, 40(1), 57-87.

American Psychiatric Association. (2013). *Diagnostic and statistical manual of mental disorders* (5th ed.). Washington, DC: Author.

Arendt-Nielsen, L. and Yarnitsky, D. (2009). Experimental and clinical applications of quantitative sensory testing applied to skin, muscles and viscera. *Journal of Pain, 10,* 556-572.

Ayres, A. J. (1964). Tactile functions: their relation to hyperactive and perceptual motor behavior. *American Journal of Occupational Therapy, 18,* 6–11.

Ayres, A. J. (1972). *Sensory integration and learning disorders.* Los Angeles: Western Psychological Services.

Baranek, G. T., David, F. J. and Poe, M. D. (2006). Sensory experience questionnaire: Discriminating sensory features in young children with autism, developmental delays, and typical development. *Journal of Child Psychology and Psychiatry, 47,* 591–601.

Barbro, B., Thermlund, G. and Nettelbladt (2006). ADHD and language impairment. *European Child and Adolescent Psychiatry, 15,* (1), 52-60.

Barbaresi, W. J., Katusic, S. K., Colligan, R. C., Pankratz, V. S., Weaver, A. L., and Weber, K. J. (2002). How common is attention-deficit/hyperactivity disorder? Incidence in a population based birth cohort in Rochester, Minn. *Archives of Pediatrics and Adolescent Medicine, 156,* 217-224.

Bar-Shalita, T., Vatine, J. and Parush, S. (2008). Sensory modulation disorder: A risk factor for participation in daily life activities. *Developmental Medicine and Child Neurology, 50* (12), 932–937.

Bar-Shalita, T., Vatine, J. J., Seltzer, Z., and Parush, S. (2009). Psychophysical correlates in children with sensory modulation disorder (SMD). *Physiology and Behavior, 98,* 631–639.

Bar-Shalita, T., Vatine, J., Yarnitsky, D., Parush, S., and Weissman-Fogel, I. (2013). Atypical central pain processing in sensory modulation disorder: Absence of temporal summation and higher after-sensation. *Experimental Brain Research.* In Press.

Barkley, R. A. (2003). Issues in the diagnosis of attention deficit/hyperactivity disorder in children. *Brain Development, 25,* 77-83.

Barkley, R. A. (2003). Issues in the diagnosis of attention deficit/hyperactivity disorder in children. *Brain and Development, 25,* 77-83.

Barkley, R. A., Murphy, K. R. and Kwasnik, D. (2006). Psychological adjustments and adaptive impairments in young adults with ADHD. *Journal of Attention Disorders, 1,* 41–54.

Ben-Sasson, A., Carter, A. S. and Briggs-Gowan, M. J. (2009). Sensory over-responsivity in elementary school: Prevalence and social-emotional correlates. *Journal of Abnormal Child Psychology, 37*(5), 705–716.

Ben-Sasson, A., Cermak, S. A., Orsmond, G. I., Carter, A. S., and Fogg, L. (2007). Can we differentiate sensory overresponsivity from anxiety symptoms in toddlers? Perspectives of occupational therapists and psychologists. *Infant Mental Health Journal, 28,* 536–558.

Ben-Sasson, A., Hen, L., Fluss, R., Cermak, S. A., Engel-Yeger, B., and Gal, E. (2009). A meta-analysis of sensory modulation symptoms in individuals with autism spectrum disorders. *Journal of Autism and Developmental Disorders, 39*(1), 1–11.

Biederman, J. and Faraone, S. V. (2005). Attention-deficit hyperactivity disorder. *Lancet, 366,* 237–248.

Brett-Green, B., Miller, L. J., Gavin, W. J., Davies, P. L. (2008). Multisensory integration in children: A preliminary ERP study. *Brain Research,* 1242, 283–290.

Brett-Green, B. A., Miller, L. J., Schoen, S. A., and Nielsen, D. M. (2010). An exploratory event related potential study of multisensory integration in sensory over-responsive children. *Brain Research,* 1321, 67-77.

Brown, T. E. (2000). Emerging understanding of attention-deficit disorders and comorbidities. In: T. E. Brown (Ed.), *Attention-deficit disorders and comorbidities in children, adolescents, and adults* (pp. 3-56). Washington, DC: American Psychiatric Press.

Brown, T. E. (2013). *A new understanding of ADHD in children and adults: Executive Function Impairments* New York, NY: Routledge.

Brown, C., Tollefson, N., Dunn, W., Cromwell, R., and Filion, D. (2001). The adult sensory profile: Measuring patterns of sensory processing. *The American Journal of Occupational Therapy,* 55, 75-82.

Byrne, J. M., Bawden, H. N., Tricia, L., Beattie, B. A., and DeWolfe, N. A. (2001). Preschoolers classified as having attention deficit hyperactivity disorder (ADHD): DSM-IV symptom endorsement pattern. *Journal of Child Neurology,* 15(8), 533-8.

Cermak, S. A. (2005). "Cognitive rehabilitation of children with attention- deficit/ hyperactivity disorder". In: *Cognition and Occupation across the Life Span,* ed. N. Katz (Bethesda, Maryland: American Occupational Therapy Association Inc.), 227-302.

Chavez, B., Sopko, M. A., Ehret, M. J., Paulino, R. E., Goldberg, K. R., Angstadt, K., et al. (2009). An update on central nervous system stimulant formulations in children and adolescents with attention-deficit/hyperactivity disorder. *The Annals of Pharmacotherapy,* 43(6), 1084–1095.

Cheung, P. P. and Siu, A. M. (2009). A comparison of patterns of sensory processing in children with and without developmental disabilities. *Research in Developmental Disabilities,* 30, 1468–1480.

Cohn, E., Miller, L. J. and Tickle-Degnen, L. (2000). Parental hopes for therapy outcomes: Children with sensory modulation disorders. *American Journal of Occupational Therapy,* 54, 36–43.

Conner, D. F., Edward, G., Fletcher, K. E., Baird, J., Barkley, R. A., and Steingard, R. J. (2003). Correlates of comorbid psychopathology in children with ADHD. *Journal of the American Academy of Child and Adolescent Psychiatry,* 42(2), 193-200.

Davies, P. L. and Gavin, W. J. (2007). Validating the diagnosis of sensory processing disorders using EEG technology. *The American Journal of Occupational Therapy,* 61, 176-189.

Davies, P. L., Chang, W. and Gavin, W. J. (2009). Maturation of sensory gating performance in children with and without sensory processing disorders. *International Journal of Psychophysiology,* 72, 187–197.

Daley, D. (2005). Attention deficit hyperactivity disorder: A review of the essential facts. *Child: Care, Health, and Development,* 32, 193–204.

De Los Reyes, A. and Kazdin, A. E. (2005). Informant discrepancies in the assessment of childhood psychopathology: A critical review, theoretical framework, and recommendations for further study. *Psychological Bulletin,* 131, 483–509.

Denckla, M. B. (2003). ADHD: Topic update. *Brain and Development,* 25(6), 383-389.

Dunn, W. (1997). The impact of sensory processing abilities on the daily lives of young Children and their families: A conceptual model. *Infants and Young Children,* 9, 3-35.

Dunn, W. (1999). *Sensory Profile's user manual.* San Antonio: TX: Psychological Corporation.

Dunn, W. (2000). Habit: what`s the brain got to do with it? *The Occupational Therapy Journal of Research,* 20, 6s- 20s.

Dunn, W. (2001). The sensations of everyday life: Empirical, theoretical, and pragmatic considerations. *American Journal of Occupational Therapy,* 55, 608-620.

Dunn, W. (2008). *Living sensationally, understanding your senses.* London, UK: Jessica Kingsley Publishers.

Dunn, W. and Bennett, D. (2002). Patterns of sensory processing in children with attention deficit hyperactivity disorder. *Occupational Therapy Journal of Research,* 22, 4-15.

Dunn, D. W. and Kronenberger, W. G. (2003). Attention deficit/hyperactivity disorder in children and adolescents. *Neurologic Clinics of North America,* 21, 933-940.

Erner, J. and Dunn, W. (1998). The Sensory Profile: A discriminant analysis of children with and without disabilities. *American Journal of Occupational Therapy,* 52, 283-290.

Faraone, S. V., Biederman, J., Spencer, T., Wilens, T., Seidman, L. J., Mick, E., and Doyle, A. E. (2000). Attention-deficit/hyperactivity disorder in adults: An overview. *Biological Psychiatry,* 48, 9–20.

Feldman, H. M. and Reiff, M. I. (2014). Attention-deficit- hyperactivity disorder in children and adolescents. *The New England Journal of Medicine,* 370, 383–846.

Fischer, M., Barkley, R. A., Smallish, L., and Fletcher, K. (2002). Young adult follow-up of hyperactive children: Self-reported psychiatric disorders, comorbidity, and the role of childhood conduct problems. *Journal of Abnormal Child Psychology,* 30, 463–475.

Fliers, E., Rommelse, N., Vermeulen, S. H. M., et al. (2008). Motor coordination problems in children and adolescents with ADHD rated by parents and teachers: effects of age and gender. *Journal of Neural Transmission,* 115(2), 211-220.

Frazier, T.W., Demarre, H.A., & Youngstrom, E.A. (2004). Meta − analysis of intellectual and neuropsychological test performance in ADHD. *Neuropsychology,* 18(3), 543-555.

Froehlich, T. E., Lanphear, B. P., Epstein, J. N., Barbaresi, W. J., Katusic, S. K., and Kahn, R. S. (2007). Prevalence, recognition, and treatment of attention-deficit/hyperactivity disorder in a national sample of US children. *Archives of Pediatrics and Adolescent Medicine,* 161(9), 857–864.

Ghanizadeh A. (2011). Sensory processing problems in children with ADHD: A systematic review. *Psychiatry Investigations* 8:89–94.

Gillberg, C. (2003). ADHD and DAMP: A general health perspective. *Child and Adolescent Mental Health,* 8(3), 106-113.

Gillberg, C., Gillberg, C. I., Rasmussen, P., Kadesjo, B., Soderstrom, H., Rastam, M., (2004). Co-existing disorders in ADHD − implications for diagnosis and intervention. *European Child and Adolescent Psychiatry,* 13(Suppl. 1), 80-92.

Gillberg, C. and Kadesjo, B. (2000). Attention-deficit/hyperactivity and developmental coordination disorder. In: T. E. Brown (Ed.), *Attention-deficit disorders and comorbidities in children, adolescents, and adults* (pp. 393-406). Washington, DC: American Psychiatric Press.

Goldsmith, H. H., Van Hulle, C. A., Arneson, C. L., Schrieber, J. E., and Gernsbacher, M. A. (2006). A population-based twin study of parentally reported tactile and auditory defensiveness in young children. *Journal of Abnormal Child Psychology,* 34, 393–407.

Gouze, K. R., Hopkins, J., Lebailly, S. A., and Lavigne, J. V. (2009). Re-examining the epidemiology of sensory regulation dysfunction and comorbid psychopathology. *Journal of Abnormal Child Psychology,* 37(8), 1077–1087.

Hanrahan, K., McCarthy, A. M., Kleiber, C., Lutgendorf, S., and Tsalikian, E. (2006). Strategies for salivary cortisol collection and analysis in research with children. *Applied Nursing Research,* 19, 95–101.

Hansson, P., Baconga, M. and Bouhassira, D. (2007). Usefulness and limitations of quantitative sensory testing: clinical and research application in neuropathic pain states. *Pain,* 129, 256-259.

Hazen, E. P., Reichert, E. L., Piacentini, J. C., Miguel, E. C., do Rosario, M. C., Pauls, D., and Geller, D. A. (2008). Case series: Sensory intolerance as a primary symptom of pediatric OCD. *Annals of Clinical Psychiatry,* 20, 199–203.

Hofmann, S. G. and Bitran, S. (2007). Sensory processing sensitivity in social anxiety disorder: Relationship to harm avoidance and diagnostic subtypes. *Journal of Anxiety Disorders,* 21, 944–954.

Interdisciplinary Council on Developmental and Learning Disorders. (2005). *Diagnostic manual for infancy and early childhood: Mental health, developmental, regulatory–sensory processing and language disorders and learning challenges (ICDL–DMIC).* Bethesda, MD: Author.

Jensen, P. S., Martin, D. and Cantwell, D. P. (1997). Comorbidity in ADHD: Implications for research, practice, and DSM-V. *Journal of the American Academy of Child and Adolescent Psychiatry,* 36, 1065–1079.

Kadesjo, B. and Gillberg, C. (2001). The comorbidity of ADHD in the general population of Swedish school-age children. *Journal of Child Psychology and Psychiatry,* 42, 487–492.

Kandel, E. R. (1991). Cellular mechanisms of learning and the biological basis of individuality. In: E. R. Kandel, J. H. Schwartz and T. M. Jessel (Eds.), *Principles of neural science* (3rd ed, pp. 1009-1031). East Norwalk, CT: Appleton and Lange.

Kessler, R. C., Green, J. G., Adler, L. A., et al. (2010). Structure and diagnosis of adult Attention-Deficit/Hyperactivity: Analysis of expanded symptom criteria from the adult ADHD clinical diagnostic scale. *Archives of General Psychiatry,* 67(11), 1168-1178.

Kinnealey, M., Oliver, B. and Wilbarger, P. (1995). A phenomenological study of sensory defensiveness in adults. *The American Journal of Occupational Therapy,* 49, 444–451.

Koziol, L. F. and Budding, D. (2012): ADHD and sensory processing disorders: Placing the diagnostic issues in context. *Applied Neuropsychology Child,* 1(2), 137-144.

Lane, S. J. (2002). Sensory modulation. In: A. C. Bundy, S. J. Lane and E. A. Murray (Eds.), *Sensory integration: Theory and practice* (2nd ed., pp. 101-122). Philadelphia: F. A. Davis Company.

Lane, S. J., Miller, L. J. and Hanft, B. E. (2000, June). Toward a consensus in terminology in sensory integration theory and practice: Part 2: Sensory integration patterns of function and dysfunction. *Sensory Integration Special Interest Section Quarterly,* 23, 1–4.

Lane, S. J., Reynolds, S. and Thacker, L. (2010). Sensory over-responsivity and ADHD: Differentiating using electrodermal responses, cortisol, and anxiety. *Frontiers in Integrative Neuroscience,* 4, 1-14.

Levy, F. (2004). Synaptic gating and ADHD: a biological theory of comorbidity of ADHD and anxiety. *Neuropsychopharmacology* 29, 1589–1596.s.

Mangeot, S. D., Miller, L. J., McIntosh, D. N., McGrath-Clarke, J., Simon, J., Hagerman, R. J., et al. (2001). Sensory modulation dysfunction in children with attention deficit hyperactivity disorder. *Developmental Medicine and Child Neurology,* 43, 399–406.

Manly, T., Robertson, I. H., Anderson, V., and Nimmo- Smith, I. (1999). *The Test of Everyday Attention for Children (TEA-Ch).* England: Thames Valley Test Company Ltd.

McIntosh, D.N., Miller, L.J., & Dunn, W (1999a). Overview of the Short Sensory Profile (SSP). In W. Dunn, (Ed.), *The sensory profile: Examiner's manual* (pp. 59–73). San Antonio: The Psychological Corporation.

McIntosh, D. N., Miller, L. J., Shyu, V., and Hagerman, R. (1999b). Sensory-modulation disruption, electrodermal responses, and functional behaviors. *Developmental Medicine and Child Neurology,* 41, 608–615.

Miller, L. J. and Lane, S. J. (2000). Toward a consensus in terminology in sensory integration theory and practice: Part 1: Taxonomy of neurophysiological processes. *Sensory Integration Special Interest Section Quarterly,* 23, 1.

Miller, L. J. (2006). *Sensational kids: Hope and help for children with sensory processing disorder (SPD).* G. P. Putnam's Sons.

Miller, L. J., Anzalone, M. E., Lane, S. J., Cermak, S. A., and Osten, E. T. (2007). Concept evolution in sensory integration: A proposed nosology for diagnosis. *The American Journal of Occupational Therapy,* 21, 135-140.

Miller, L. J., Coll, J. R. and Schoen, S. A. (2007). A randomized controlled pilot study of the effectiveness of occupational therapy for children with sensory modulation disorder. *The American Journal of Occupational Therapy,* 61(2), 228–238.

Miller, L. J., Nielsen, D. M. and Schoen, S. A. (2012). Attention deficit hyperactivity disorder and sensory modulation disorder: A comparison of behavior and physiology. *Research in Developmental Disabilities,* 33, 804–818.

Miller, L. J., Reisman, J. E., McIntosh, D. N., and Simon, J. (2001). An ecological model of sensory modulation: Performance of children with Fragile X syndrome, autism, attention-deficit/hyperactivity disorder, and sensory modulation dysfunction. In: S. S. Roley, E. I. Blanche and R. C. Schaaf (Eds.), *Understanding the nature of sensory integration with diverse populations* (pp. 57–88). San Antonio, TX: Therapy Skill Builders.

Morrell, J. and Murray, L. (2003). Parenting and the development of conduct disorder and hyperactive symptoms in childhood: A prospective longitudinal study from 2 months to 8 years. *Journal of Child Psychology and Psychiatry,* 44, 489-508.

Nigg, J. T. (2005). Neuropsychologic theory and findings in attention deficit/hyperactivity disorder: The state of the field and salient challenges for the coming decade. *Biological Psychiatry,* 57, 1424-1435.

Nigg, J. T. (2006). Temperament and developmental psychopathology. *Journal of Child Psychology and Psychiatry,* 47, 395–422.

Ognibene, T. C. (2002). *Distinguishing sensory modulation dysfunction from attention deficit hyperactivity disorder: Sensory habituation and response inhibition processes.* University of Denver, Faculty of Social Sciences: Unpublished dissertations.

Owen, J. P., Marco, E. J., Desai, S., Fourie, E., Harris, J., Hill, S. S., Arnett, A. B., and Mukherjee, P. (2013). Abnormal white matter microstructure in children with sensory processing disorders. *NeuroImage: Clinical,* 2, 844-853.

Parham, L. D. and Johnson-Ecker, C. (2002). "Evaluation of sensory processing: research version 4", In: *Sensory Integration: Theory and Practice* (2nd ed.), eds. A. C. Bundy, S. J. Lane and E. A. Murray, (Philadelphia: F. A. Davis), 194-196.

Parham, L. D. and Mailloux, Z. (1996). Sensory integration. In: J. Case-Smith, A. S. Allen and P. N. Pratt (Eds.), *Occupational therapy for children* (3rd ed., pp. 307-355). St. Louis: Mosby-Year Book, Inc.

Parush, S., Sohmer, H., Steinberg, A., and Kaitz, M. (1997). Somatosensory processing in children with attention deficit hyperactivity disorder. *Developmental Medicine and Child Neurology,* 39, 464-468.

Parush, P., Sohmer, H., Steinberg, A., and Kaitz, M. (2007). Somatosensory function in boys with ADHD and tactile defensiveness. *Physiology and Behavior,* 90, 553-558.

Pfeiffer, B., Daly, B.P., Nicholls, E.G., and Gullo, D.F. (2014). Assessing sensory processing problems in children with and without Attention Deficit Hyperactivity Disorder. *Physical & Occupational Therapy in Pediatrics*, DOI: 10.3109/01942638.2014.904471.

Pierce, K. (2003). Attention-deficit/hyperactivity disorder and comorbidity. *Primary Psychiatry,* 10(4), 69 - 76.

Pliszka, S. R. (1998). Comorbidity of attention-deficit/hyperactivity disorder with psychiatric disorder: An overview. *Journal of Clinical Psychiatry*, 59(Suppl. 7), 50-58.

Reeves, G. D. (2001). From neuron to behavior: regulation, arousal and attention as important substrates for the process of sensory integration. In: S. S. Roley, E. I. Blanche and R. C. Schaaf (Eds.), *Understanding the nature of sensory integration with diverse populations* (pp. 57–88). San Antonio, TX: Therapy Skill Builders.

Reynolds, S., Lane, S. J. (2008). Diagnostic validity of sensory over-responsivity: A review of the literature and case reports. *Journal of Autism and Developmental Disorders,* 38, 516-529.

Reynolds, S., Lane, S. J. and Gennings, C. (2009). The moderating role of sensory over-responsivity in HPA activity: a pilot study with children diagnosed with ADHD. *Journal of Attention Disorders,* 13, 468-478.

Robison, L. M., Sclar, D. A., Skaer, T. L., and Galin, R. S. (2004). Treatment modalities among US children diagnosed with ADHD. 1995-1999. *International Clinical Psychopharmacology, 19,* 17-22.

Roid, G. H. and Miller, L. J. (1997). *Leiter International Performance Scale—Revised.* Wood Dale, IL: Stoelting Company.

Rutter, M. and Silberg, J. (2002). Gene-environment interplay in relation to emotional and behavioral disturbance. *Annual Review of Psychology,* 53, 463-490.

Schaaf, R. C., Miller, L. J., Seawell, D., and O'Keefe, S. (2003). Children with disturbances in sensory processing: A pilot study examining the role of the parasympathetic nervous system. *American Journal of Occupational Therapy,* 57, 442–449.

Sonuga-Barke, E. J. S., Auerbach, J., Campbell, S. B., Daley, D., and Thompson, M. (2005). Varieties of preschool hyperactivity: Multiple pathways from risk to disorder. *Developmental Science*, 8(2), 141-150.

Swanson, J. M. (1992). *School based assessments and interventions for ADD students.* Irvine, CA: KC Publications.

Tseng, M. H., Henderson, A., Chow, S. M. K., and Yao, G. (2004). Relationship between motor proficiency, attention, impulse and activity in children with ADHD. *Developmental Medicine and Child Neurology,* 46(6), 381-390.

Van Hulle, C. A., Schmidt, N. L. and Goldsmith, H. H. (2012). Is sensory over-responsivity distinguishable from childhood behavior problems? A phenotypic and genetic analysis. *Journal of Child Psychology and Psychiatry,* 53, 64-72.

Verdugo, R. and Ochoa, J. L. (1992). Quantitative somatosensory thermotest. A key method for functional evaluation of small caliber afferent channels. *Brain,* 115, 893-913.

Wassenberg, R., Hendriksen, J. G. M., Hurks, P. P. M., et al. (2010). Speed of Language Comprehension is Impaired in ADHD. *Journal of Attention Disorders* (13) 374-385.

Wehmeier, P. M., Schacht, A., Barkley, R. A. (2010). Social and Emotional Impairment in Children and Adolescents with ADHD and the Impact on Quality of Life. *Journal of Adolescent Health,* 46, 209-217.

WHO (World Health Organization) (2001). *International Classification of Functioning, Disability and Health.* Geneva: World Health Organization.

Yochman, A., Parush, S., and Ornoy, A. (2004). Responses of Preschool Children with and without ADHD to Sensory Events in Daily Life. *American Journal of Occupational Therapy,* 58, 294-302.

Yochman, A., Ornoy, A. and Parush, S. (2006). Co-occurrence of developmental delays among preschool children with attention-deficit-hyperactivity disorder. *Developmental Medicine and Child Disorder,* 48, 483-488.

Yochman, A., Alon-Beery, O., Sribman, A., and Parush, S. (2013). Differential diagnosis of sensory modulation dysfunction (SMD) and attention deficit hyperactivity disorder (ADHD): Participation, sensation, and attention. *Frontiers in Human Neuroscience*, 7, 1-10.

Zero to Three. (2005). *Diagnostic classification: 0-3R: Diagnostic classification of mental health and developmental disorders in infancy and early childhood (Revised ed.).* Washington, DC: Zero to Three Press.

In: ADHD
Editors: Itai Berger and Adina Maeir
ISBN: 978-1-63321-047-9
© 2014 Nova Science Publishers, Inc.

Chapter 5

INTRAUTERINE GROWTH RETARDATION AND ADHD

Noa Ofek-Shlomai, M.D.[*]

Department of Neonatology,
Hadassah-Hebrew University Medical Center, Jerusalem, Israel

ABSTRACT

Introduction: Intrauterine growth retardation (IUGR) is a reduction from expected fetal growth patterns. IUGR may be associated with innate fetal or placental issues. The hypothesis of developmental origins of health and disease consists of the idea that structure and functions of cells and organs may be influenced by adverse influences during susceptible periods of development. The consequences of programming may include both adult health and disease states, and behavioral patterns. ADHD is considered more prevalent in ex-preterm and growth restricted children. Pathophysiological theories include:

I   Reduced carbohydrate and protein in late pregnancy is associated with IUGR and animal models demonstrated an effect on dopamine related behaviors such as reward processing and hyperactivity.

II In asymmetric IUGR infants, the head circumference is relatively preserved due to a physiologic adaptation process. Brain sparing is important for neonatal survival without major neurodevelopmental impairment, but may not be sufficient to fully compensate for aberrant cellular successions. Studies show structural alterations in IUGR infants, consisting of a reduction in intracranial volume and cortical gray matter. ADHD was reported to be associated with decreased total brain volume.

III The fetus may be exposed to glucocorticoids during maternal stress, or via synthetic provision. This may cause lower birth weight, increased infant activity of the hypothalamic-pituitary- adrenocortical axis and hyperactivity.

Numerous studies have shown an association between ADHD and prematurity, low and very low birth weight and IUGR. Animal models demonstrated neurobehavioral testing shows significantly higher degrees of anxiety, attention and memory problems in

---

[*] Correspondence: Noa Ofek-Shlomai, M.D. Department of Neonatology, Hadassah-Hebrew University Medical Center, Jerusalem, Israel, E-mail: noaofek@hadassah.org.il

IUGR rabbit pups, and Connectivity analysis revealed lower ratios of fibers within the networks correlating with functional outcomes.

A study of 123 IUGR infants, matched with 63 infants followed up for 9 years reported ex-IUGR infants to have more neuropsychological difficulties, including general cognitive competence and specific neuropsychological skills.

Another study reported higher mean scores in IUGR preterm group compared to AGA preterm and term controls, in the subtests that addressed behavior deviance and ADHD scores. Additional studies support these results.

Conclusion: intrauterine growth restriction has a significant effect on future neurodevelopment of term and preterm infants. Animal models, imaging and clinical research support this conclusion. ADHD in ex-IUGR children may have a unique phenotype.

DEFINITIONS

Intrauterine growth retardation (IUGR) is a reduction from expected fetal growth patterns. IUGR is the result of any process that inhibits fetal growth and can be associated with innate fetal or placental issues [1, 2]. Fetal causes, such as viral infections, genetic factors and maternal under nutrition in early pregnancy [3] usually result in long term IUGR causing proportionate reductions in weight, length and head circumference (*symmetric IUGR*). These infants have a normal ponderal index (kg/m^3). Uteroplacental vascular insufficiency, which is often short term, tends to cause *asymmetric IUGR*, with subnormal weight and near normal head circumference and length and thus a low ponderal index [1]

Small for gestational age (SGA) infants are infants whose weight is lower than population norms or lower than a predetermined cutoff (e.g., -2SD, <5th or 10th percentile). The cause may be pathological (such as IUGR) or nonpathological such as smaller ethnically derived growth curves or individual growth potential. Not all SGA infants are therefore intrauterine growth restricted [1, 3].

For the scope of this chapter, we will concentrate on the association between IUGR and ADHD.

PATHOPHYSIOLOGY

The hypothesis of developmental origins of health and disease was introduced by Gillman et al. in 2005 [4, 5]. According to this hypothesis, structure and functions of cells and organs may be influenced by adverse influences during susceptible periods of development. These function changes may persist throughout life [5, 6]. The consequences of programming include both adult health and disease states, and a wide range of behavioral patterns that may manifest in childhood [7]. Externalizing disorders such as ADHD and associated problems and symptoms are of particular interest in this context. ADHD is considered a multifaceted, including genetic [4, 8] and pre and post natal environmental influences [9, 10].

Pathophysiology of ADHD is thought to involve prefrontal and striatal dysfunctional dopaminergic and noroadrenaline neurotransmission [11, 12].

It has been reported that IUGR, particularly asymmetrical IUGR, is associated with ADHD. The processes that may influence this neurodevelopmental programing include:

Maternal macronutrient intake: Moore et al. [13] reported reduced carbohydrate and protein in late pregnancy was associated in lower ponderal index in the offspring. In a study conducted by Vucetic et al. [14] mouse dams were fed a protein restricted (8.5%) or an isocaloric (18% protein) diet throughout pregnancy and lactation (a validated rodent model of IUGR). IUGR offspring had a 6-8 overexpression of dopamine related genes. These animals demonstrated alternations in dopamine related behaviors such as reward processing and hyperactivity [14]. This effect of maternal macronutrient intake on ADHD may point to a potentially modifiable element in the pathophysiology of ADHD [4].

Brain sparing processes and brain growth: in asymmetric IUGR infants, the head circumference is relatively preserved due to a physiologic adaptation process which includes redistribution of blood flow which is directed to the brain [15]. This results in accelerated neuromaturation, which improves survival outcome, but the consequence of that compensatory mechanism may be poorer cognitive outcome [16]. Brain sparing is important for neonatal survival without major neurodevelopmental impairment, but may not be sufficient to fully compensate for aberrant cellular successions and the altered neurodevelopmental route associated with them. Tolsa et al. [17] reported structural alterations in IUGR infants, consisting of a significant reduction in intracranial volume and cortical gray matter [17]. In view of the limitations of brain sparing processes, selective cortical vulnerability is expected. Data alludes to increased susceptibility of hippocampal structures, limbic structures and the frontal lobe [18, 19]. This may suggest a typical neuropsychological profile including "soft" neurological symptoms such as learning and behavioral difficulties, including ADHD [20-27].

Glucocoticoids: the fetus may be exposed to glucorticoids during maternal psychological or physiological stress, as well as via synthetic provision of steroids. This may cause lower birth weight [28, 29], increased infant activity of the hypothalamic-pituitary- adrenocortical axis and hyperactivity [28, 30], and a preferential decrease in brain growth [29]. ADHD was reported to be associated with decreased total brain volume [31]. However, The ratio of corpus striatum volume to brain volume did not correlate with the degree of IUGR in a study conducted by Toft et al. [32].

Furthermore, studies in rodents have shown prenatal exposure to synthetic glucocorticoids alter dopamine and noradrenaline neurotransmission [33]. Lindely et al. [34] reported inhibition of dopamine metabolism in adult rats treated with glucocorticosteroids.

Lactate: in a study of preterm, term and IUGR infants, significant higher lactate levels were found in infants with IUGR [35]. This less favorable metabolic state may interfere to some extent with the synaptic organization of the striatal circuits, or may be interpreted as a result of delayed striatal development [36].

EVIDENCE FOR AN ASSOCIATION BETWEEN ADHD AND IUGR

Numerous studies have shown an association between ADHD and prematurity, low and very low birth weight and IUGR [2, 4, 20, 37-39].

Illa et al. [40] explored the long term functional outcomes and correlation with regional brain connectivity by MRI diffusion tractography metrics in near term rabbit model of IUGR. The rabbit pups were delivered at 30 days of gestation and were functionally evaluated by open field behavioral tests, which evaluate anxiety, attention and object recognition. Subsequently, brains were collected, fixated and high resolution MRI was performed. The authors reported cognitive and neurobehavioral testing showed significantly higher degrees of anxiety, attention and memory problems in IUGR cases compared to AGA controls. Analysis revealed significant differences between groups in multiple brain regions, mostly grey matter structures. Connectivity analysis revealed lower ratios of fibers within the networks in cases vs. controls. These results correlated with functional outcomes [40].

Geva et al. [20] conducted a study of 123 IUGR infants, matched with 63 infants for gestational age and socioeconomical factors followed up for 9 years.

The experimental group was matched at 9 years of age with a group of 63 children selected from the same community in the Tel Aviv municipal area. The groups were matched for testing age, parental ages, maternal education, parental occupation, and gestational age. At 9 years of age, the participants were evaluated with an extensive neuropsychological testing battery. The testing battery included estimation of cognitive abilities using 2 methods: (1) a 2-test short form of the Wechsler tests of intelligence-revised [41, 42] and (2) the Goodenough-Harris Draw-A-Person test [43]. Academic achievements were evaluated by the achievement scale tests of the Kaufmann Assessment Battery for Children [44]; learning and memory skills by the Rey-Osterrieth Complex Rey Auditory Verbal Learning Test [45] and the Visual Auditory Digit Span Evaluation [46]; attention and executive functions using selected subtests of the Neuropsycholological Evaluation for Children [47]. They reported ex-IUGR infants to have more neuropsychological difficulties. These included general cognitive competence as well as specific neuropsychological skills such as visuomotor integration, language and executive functions [20]. These findings point to frontal lobe related suboptimal development.

Morsing et al. [38] compared full term, appropriate for gestational age (AGA) preterm and IUGR preterm infants. Cognitive evaluation was performed on 102 children at 5 to 8 years of chronological age. Matched children were examined at an age within 2 months of the index children. Wechsler Preschool and Primary Scale of Intelligence-III were used. The parents were interviewed and filled in scoring questionnaires regarding prevalence of attention-deficit disorder using Brown's ADD scales [48]. Brown's ADD questionnaire consists of 44 items and examines the ability to sustain attention, activate and organize work tasks, sustain energy and effort to complete tasks, regulate moods, use short-term working memory, and recall learned material. A summary score of >55 was considered to indicate attention and deficit disorders. For behavioral problems the Strengths and Difficulties Questionnaire (SDQ) was used [49]. The authors found no difference between AGA term and preterm infants in behavioral and ADHD scores. They reported higher mean scores in the IUGR preterm group in the SDQ [49] subtests that addressed behavior deviance and ADHD scores. Boys from the preterm IUGR group had significantly lower verbal and full scale IQ while no correlating difference was found in girls from the same group [38].

In a prospective study Walther et al. [2] compared 25 asymmetrical IUGR consecutive infants to 25 AGA infants up to 7 years of age. Teachers were contacted when the child had reached the age of 7 years. They completed a questionnaire including behavioral and academic characteristics. The behavioral items examined were: (1) activity, (2) shyness and withdrawal, (3) concentration, (4) difficulty in managing, (5) temper tantrums, (6) relations with other children, (7) irritability, (8) fears, (9) destruction and aggression and (10) clumsiness. The academic items examined were: (1) cognitive development, (2) social skills and (3) motor skills. The score of each child was summed and all items were also analyzed separately. The authors reported more neurological dysfunction and problematic behavior in the growth restricted infants. This was especially evident in hyperactivity, poor concentration, clumsiness, fears and language delay. Overall academic achievements also showed a disadvantage for growth-restricted infants [2].

A population-based study of 5181 English children AGED 4-15 demonstrated a linear association between lower birth weight and higher scores on the hyperactivity subscale of the SDQ [49] for boys, and peer problems in girls. These results remained intact after adjusting for social class [39].

In 2006 Lahti et al. [4] performed a study aimed at testing if among healthy full-term infants, low birth weight, length, ponderal index and head circumference to length ratio are predictive for behavioral symptoms of ADHD at the age of 5-6 years. The study population included 267 mother-father-child triads. Behavioral symptoms of ADHD were rated by the mother and the father of the child on the ADHD Rating Scale [50] at the age of five to six years. The scale consists of 14 items directly adapted from the ADHD symptoms list in the Diagnostic and Statistical Manual of Mental Disorders 3rd edition [52]. Each item is rated on a four-point scale ranging from 'Does not describe my child at all' [50] to 'Describes my child very well' [3]. The items are then summed, a higher total score indicating that ADHD symptoms are more descriptive of the child's behavior. They found that lower weight and length, and smaller head circumference, ponderal index and head circumference to length ratios predicted significantly higher total, and inattention-hyperactivity subscale scores on the ADHD rating scale. Multivariate analysis adjusting for gender, socioeconomic factors etc. did not change these results [4].

Klaric et al. [52] 50 IUGR full term infants and compares their neuropsycholgical development at preschool age to 50 AGA infants born in the same time period. Biometric parameters collected for both groups of children were birth weight, head circumference, current body weight, and current head circumference. Neurological development was evaluated by the Touwen neurological examination [53]. Cognitive development was assessed using the C˘ uturic´ developmental test [52], and imitative hand positions, and a visual attention test were evaluated using a Developmental Neuropsychological Assessment [47]. The authors reported fine motor skills were the most significant difference between groups. However, when analyzing by postnatal head growth and comparing ex growth restricted preschoolers with head circumference <10 percentile to those >10 percentile, the found marginally significant differences in developmental aspects and visual attention [52].

Studies suggest that very low birth weight (VLBW) children are at increased risk for ADHD [54-62]. Strang-Karlson et al. [37] studied weather this effect differed between IUGR VLBW infants and AGA infants. The study included 52 IUGR VLBW infants' and 110 AGA infants compared to 172 term comparison subjects. Behavioral symptoms of ADHD were evaluated by a psychological questionnaire, the Adult Problem Questionnaire [63], which measures behavioral symptoms of ADHD. The questionnaire was conducted at young adulthood. Risk-taking behavior was operationalized in terms of substance use. Each participant completed a questionnaire inquiring about alcohol use (quantity and frequency of use and frequency of becoming drunk) and use of tobacco.

The authors reported IUGR VLBW young adults scored higher on executive dysfunction and emotional instability than AGA peers and control term subjects. In this group there was a more even distribution between male and female than in general population ADHD, less hyperactivity in relatively to inattention and less risk taking behavior, suggestion a distinct phenotype of ADHD in this group. The authors concluded that IUGR is a greater predictor for future ADHD than prematurity and VLBW per se [37].

In conclusion, intrauterine growth restriction may have a significant effect on future neurodevelopment of term and preterm infants. Motor impairments include fine motor skills, impairment of spatial orientation, coordination, graphomotor skills, balance and hypotonia [24, 52, 64]. Cognitive impairments include lower intelligence, creativity and executive function disorders, working and short term memory deficits, visumotor and visuspatial impairments as well as behavioral difficulties and ADHD [51, 65, 66].

REFERENCES

[1]   Martin R.J FAA, Walsh MC. *Neonatal-Perinatal Medicine.* 8th ed. Philadelphia, USA: Mosby Elsevier; 2006.

[2]   Walther FJ. Growth and development of term disproportionate small-for-gestational age infants at the age of 7 years. *Early human development.* 1988;18(1):1-11. Epub 1988/11/01.

[3]   Villar J, Belizan JM. The timing factor in the pathophysiology of the intrauterine growth retardation syndrome. *Obstetrical & gynecological survey.* 1982;37(8):499-506. Epub 1982/08/01.

[4]   Lahti J, Raikkonen K, Kajantie E, Heinonen K, Pesonen AK, Jarvenpaa AL, et al. Small body size at birth and behavioural symptoms of ADHD in children aged five to six years. *Journal of child psychology and psychiatry, and allied disciplines.* 2006;47(11):1167-74. Epub 2006/11/02.

[5]   Gillman MW. Developmental origins of health and disease. *The New England journal of medicine.* 2005;353(17):1848-50. Epub 2005/10/28.

[6]   Barker DJ. Intrauterine programming of coronary heart disease and stroke. *Acta Paediatr Suppl.* 1997;423:178-82; discussion 83. Epub 1997/12/24.

[7]   van Os J, Wichers M, Danckaerts M, Van Gestel S, Derom C, Vlietinck R. A prospective twin study of birth weight discordance and child problem behavior. *Biological psychiatry.* 2001;50(8):593-9. Epub 2001/11/03.

[8]   Faraone SV, Perlis RH, Doyle AE, Smoller JW, Goralnick JJ, Holmgren MA, et al. Molecular genetics of attention-deficit/hyperactivity disorder. *Biological psychiatry.* 2005;57(11):1313-23. Epub 2005/06/14.

[9]   Linnet KM, Dalsgaard S, Obel C, Wisborg K, Henriksen TB, Rodriguez A, et al. Maternal lifestyle factors in pregnancy risk of attention deficit hyperactivity disorder and associated behaviors: review of the current evidence. *The American journal of psychiatry.* 2003;160(6):1028-40. Epub 2003/06/05.

[10]   Morrell J, Murray L. Parenting and the development of conduct disorder and hyperactive symptoms in childhood: a prospective longitudinal study from 2 months to

8 years. *Journal of child psychology and psychiatry, and allied disciplines.* 2003;44(4):489-508. Epub 2003/05/20.

[11] Castellanos FX. Toward a pathophysiology of attention-deficit/hyperactivity disorder. *Clinical pediatrics.* 1997;36(7):381-93. Epub 1997/07/01.

[12] Davids E, Zhang K, Tarazi FI, Baldessarini RJ. Animal models of attention-deficit hyperactivity disorder. *Brain research Brain research reviews.* 2003;42(1):1-21. Epub 2003/04/02.

[13] Moore VM, Davies MJ, Willson KJ, Worsley A, Robinson JS. Dietary composition of pregnant women is related to size of the baby at birth. *The Journal of nutrition.* 2004;134(7):1820-6. Epub 2004/07/01.

[14] Vucetic Z, Totoki K, Schoch H, Whitaker KW, Hill-Smith T, Lucki I, et al. Early life protein restriction alters dopamine circuitry. *Neuroscience.* 2010;168(2):359-70. Epub 2010/04/17.

[15] Inder TE, Wells SJ, Mogridge NB, Spencer C, Volpe JJ. Defining the nature of the cerebral abnormalities in the premature infant: a qualitative magnetic resonance imaging study. *The Journal of pediatrics.* 2003;143(2):171-9. Epub 2003/09/13.

[16] Scherjon SA, Oosting H, Smolders-DeHaas H, Zondervan HA, Kok JH. Neurodevelopmental outcome at three years of age after fetal 'brain-sparing'. *Early human development.* 1998;52(1):67-79. Epub 1998/10/03.

[17] Tolsa CB, Zimine S, Warfield SK, Freschi M, Sancho Rossignol A, Lazeyras F, et al. Early alteration of structural and functional brain development in premature infants born with intrauterine growth restriction. *Pediatric research.* 2004;56(1):132-8. Epub 2004/05/07.

[18] Nyakas C, Buwalda B, Luiten PG. Hypoxia and brain development. *Progress in neurobiology.* 1996;49(1):1-51. Epub 1996/05/01.

[19] Lingas R, Dean F, Matthews SG. Maternal nutrient restriction (48 h) modifies brain corticosteroid receptor expression and endocrine function in the fetal guinea pig. *Brain research.* 1999;846(2):236-42. Epub 1999/11/11.

[20] Geva R, Eshel R, Leitner Y, Valevski AF, Harel S. Neuropsychological outcome of children with intrauterine growth restriction: a 9-year prospective study. *Pediatrics.* 2006;118(1):91-100. Epub 2006/07/05.

[21] Low JA, Handley-Derry MH, Burke SO, Peters RD, Pater EA, Killen HL, et al. Association of intrauterine fetal growth retardation and learning deficits at age 9 to 11 years. *American journal of obstetrics and gynecology.* 1992;167(6):1499-505. Epub 1992/12/01.

[22] Goyen TA, Veddovi M, Lui K. Developmental outcome of discordant premature twins at 3 years. *Early human development.* 2003;73(1-2):27-37. Epub 2003/08/23.

[23] Janvier A, Khairy M, Kokkotis A, Cormier C, Messmer D, Barrington KJ. Apnea is associated with neurodevelopmental impairment in very low birth weight infants. *Journal of perinatology : official journal of the California Perinatal Association.* 2004;24(12):763-8. Epub 2004/08/27.

[24] Leitner Y, Fattal-Valevski A, Geva R, Bassan H, Posner E, Kutai M, et al. Six-year follow-up of children with intrauterine growth retardation: long-term, prospective study. *Journal of child neurology.* 2000;15(12):781-6. Epub 2001/02/24.

[25] O'Keeffe MJ, O'Callaghan M, Williams GM, Najman JM, Bor W. Learning, cognitive, and attentional problems in adolescents born small for gestational age. *Pediatrics.* 2003;112(2):301-7. Epub 2003/08/05.

[26] Larroque B, Bertrais S, Czernichow P, Leger J. School difficulties in 20-year-olds who were born small for gestational age at term in a regional cohort study. *Pediatrics.* 2001;108(1):111-5. Epub 2001/07/04.

[27] Zubrick SR, Kurinczuk JJ, McDermott BM, McKelvey RS, Silburn SR, Davies LC. Fetal growth and subsequent mental health problems in children aged 4 to 13 years. *Developmental medicine and child neurology.* 2000;42(1):14-20. Epub 2000/02/09.

[28] French NP, Hagan R, Evans SF, Godfrey M, Newnham JP. Repeated antenatal corticosteroids: size at birth and subsequent development. *American journal of obstetrics and gynecology.* 1999;180(1 Pt 1):114-21. Epub 1999/01/23.

[29] Thorp JA, Jones PG, Peabody JL, Knox E, Clark RH. Effect of antenatal and postnatal corticosteroid therapy on weight gain and head circumference growth in the nursery. *Obstetrics and gynecology.* 2002;99(1):109-15. Epub 2002/01/05.

[30] Matthews SG. Antenatal glucocorticoids and programming of the developing CNS. *Pediatric research.* 2000;47(3):291-300. Epub 2000/03/10.

[31] Krain AL, Castellanos FX. Brain development and ADHD. *Clinical psychology review.* 2006;26(4):433-44. Epub 2006/02/17.

[32] Toft PB, Leth H, Ring PB, Peitersen B, Lou HC, Henriksen O. Volumetric analysis of the normal infant brain and in intrauterine growth retardation. *Early human development.* 1995;43(1):15-29. Epub 1995/08/30.

[33] Muneoka K, Mikuni M, Ogawa T, Kitera K, Kamei K, Takigawa M, et al. Prenatal dexamethasone exposure alters brain monoamine metabolism and adrenocortical response in rat offspring. *The American journal of physiology.* 1997;273(5 Pt 2):R1669-75. Epub 1997/12/31.

[34] Lindley SE, Bengoechea TG, Schatzberg AF, Wong DL. Glucocorticoid effects on mesotelencephalic dopamine neurotransmission. *Neuropsychopharmacology : official publication of the American College of Neuropsychopharmacology.* 1999;21(3):399-407. Epub 1999/08/24.

[35] Leth H, Toft PB, Pryds O, Peitersen B, Lou HC, Henriksen O. Brain lactate in preterm and growth-retarded neonates. *Acta Paediatr.* 1995;84(5):495-9. Epub 1995/05/01.

[36] Toft PB. Prenatal and perinatal striatal injury: a hypothetical cause of attention-deficit-hyperactivity disorder? *Pediatric neurology.* 1999;21(3):602-10. Epub 1999/10/08.

[37] Strang-Karlsson S, Raikkonen K, Pesonen AK, Kajantie E, Paavonen EJ, Lahti J, et al. Very low birth weight and behavioral symptoms of attention deficit hyperactivity disorder in young adulthood: the Helsinki study of very-low-birth-weight adults. *The American journal of psychiatry.* 2008;165(10):1345-53. Epub 2008/07/17.

[38] Morsing E, Asard M, Ley D, Stjernqvist K, Marsal K. Cognitive function after intrauterine growth restriction and very preterm birth. *Pediatrics.* 2011;127(4):e874-82. Epub 2011/03/09.

[39] Kelly YJ, Nazroo JY, McMunn A, Boreham R, Marmot M. Birthweight and behavioural problems in children: a modifiable effect? *International journal of epidemiology.* 2001;30(1):88-94. Epub 2001/02/15.

[40] Illa M, Eixarch E, Batalle D, Arbat-Plana A, Munoz-Moreno E, Figueras F, et al. Long-term functional outcomes and correlation with regional brain connectivity by MRI

diffusion tractography metrics in a near-term rabbit model of intrauterine growth restriction. *PloS one.* 2013;8(10):e76453. Epub 2013/10/22.

[41] Wechsler D. *Wechsler scales of intelligence.* Jerusalem, Israel: Ministry of Education; 1998.

[42] Ryan JJ, Utley AP, Worthen VE. Comparison of two IQ conversion tables for the Vocabulary-Block Design short form. *Journal of clinical psychology.* 1988;44(6):950-2. Epub 1988/11/01.

[43] ter Laak J, de Goede M, Aleva A, van Rijswijk P. The Draw-A-Person Test: an indicator of children's cognitive and socioemotional adaptation? *The Journal of genetic psychology.* 2005;166(1):77-93. Epub 2005/03/24.

[44] Kauffman AS. Assesment battery for children. In: *Education Mo*, editor. Jerusalem, Israel1996.

[45] Vakil E, Blachstein H, Rochberg J, Vardi M. Characterization of memory impairment following closed-head injury in children using the Rey Auditory Verbal Learning Test (AVLT). *Child neuropsychology : a journal on normal and abnormal development in childhood and adolescence.* 2004;10(2):57-66. Epub 2004/12/14.

[46] Koppitz EM. The visual aural digit span test for seventh graders: a normative study. *Journal of learning disabilities.* 1981;14(2):93-5. Epub 1981/02/01.

[47] Korkman M KV, Kemp S. NEPS- A Developmental neuropsychological assessment. *The Psychology Cooppration;* San Antonio, TX1998.

[48] T B. Brown attention deficit disorder scale for children and adolecsents. *The Psychological Cooporation*; San Antonio, TX2003.

[49] Goodman R. The Strengths and Difficulties Questionnaire: a research note. Journal of child psychology and psychiatry, and allied disciplines. 1997;38(5):581-6. Epub 1997/07/01.

[50] DuPaul GJ. *Parent and teacher ratings of ADHD symptoms: Psychometric properties in a community-based sample1991.* 245 p.

[51] *Diagnostic and statistical manual of mental disorders.* 3rd ed. Association AP, editor. Washington D.C, usa1987.

[52] Klaric AS, Galic S, Kolundzic Z, Bosnjak VM. Neuropsychological development in preschool children born with asymmetrical intrauterine growth restriction and impact of postnatal head growth. *Journal of child neurology.* 2013;28(7):867-73. Epub 2012/08/24.

[53] B.C.L T. *Examination of the child with minor neurological dysfunction. london,* UK1979.

[54] Saigal S, Doyle LW. An overview of mortality and sequelae of preterm birth from infancy to adulthood. *Lancet.* 2008;371(9608):261-9. Epub 2008/01/22.

[55] Hack M, Youngstrom EA, Cartar L, Schluchter M, Taylor HG, Flannery D, et al. *Behavioral outcomes and evidence of psychopathology among very low birth weight infants at age 20 years. Pediatrics.* 2004;114(4):932-40. Epub 2004/10/07.

[56] Bhutta AT, Cleves MA, Casey PH, Cradock MM, Anand KJ. Cognitive and behavioral outcomes of school-aged children who were born preterm: a meta-analysis. *JAMA : the journal of the American Medical Association.* 2002;288(6):728-37. Epub 2002/08/10.

[57] Levy-Shiff R, Einat G, Mogilner MB, Lerman M, Krikler R. Biological and environmental correlates of developmental outcome of prematurely born infants in

early adolescence. *Journal of pediatric psychology.* 1994;19(1):63-78. Epub 1994/02/01.

[58] Elgen I, Sommerfelt K, Markestad T. Population based, controlled study of behavioural problems and psychiatric disorders in low birthweight children at 11 years of age. *Archives of disease in childhood Fetal and neonatal edition.* 2002;87(2):F128-32. Epub 2002/08/24.

[59] Botting N, Powls A, Cooke RW, Marlow N. Attention deficit hyperactivity disorders and other psychiatric outcomes in very low birthweight children at 12 years. *Journal of child psychology and psychiatry, and allied disciplines.* 1997;38(8):931-41. Epub 1997/12/31.

[60] Indredavik MS, Vik T, Heyerdahl S, Kulseng S, Fayers P, Brubakk AM. Psychiatric symptoms and disorders in adolescents with low birth weight. *Archives of disease in childhood Fetal and neonatal edition.* 2004;89(5):F445-50. Epub 2004/08/24.

[61] Saigal S, Pinelli J, Hoult L, Kim MM, Boyle M. Psychopathology and social competencies of adolescents who were extremely low birth weight. *Pediatrics.* 2003;111(5 Pt 1):969-75. Epub 2003/05/03.

[62] Dahl LB, Kaaresen PI, Tunby J, Handegard BH, Kvernmo S, Ronning JA. Emotional, behavioral, social, and academic outcomes in adolescents born with very low birth weight. *Pediatrics.* 2006;118(2):e449-59. Epub 2006/08/03.

[63] Beck AT, Ward CH, Mendelson M, Mock J, Erbaugh J. An inventory for measuring depression. *Archives of general psychiatry.* 1961;4:561-71. Epub 1961/06/01.

[64] Leitner Y, Fattal-Valevski A, Geva R, Eshel R, Toledano-Alhadef H, Rotstein M, et al. Neurodevelopmental outcome of children with intrauterine growth retardation: a longitudinal, 10-year prospective study. *Journal of child neurology.* 2007;22(5):580-7. Epub 2007/08/11.

[65] Yanney M, Marlow N. Paediatric consequences of fetal growth restriction. *Seminars in fetal & neonatal medicine.* 2004;9(5):411-8. Epub 2005/02/05.

[66] Guellec I, Lapillonne A, Renolleau S, Charlaluk ML, Roze JC, Marret S, et al. Neurologic outcomes at school age in very preterm infants born with severe or mild growth restriction. *Pediatrics.* 2011;127(4):e883-91. Epub 2011/03/09.

In: ADHD
Editors: Itai Berger and Adina Maeir

ISBN: 978-1-63321-047-9
© 2014 Nova Science Publishers, Inc.

Chapter 6

COGNITIVE FUNCTIONAL (COG-FUN) INTERVENTION FOR CHILDREN WITH ADHD: THEORY AND PRACTICE

Adina Maeir[*], *Ph.D., Jeri Hahn-Markowitz, Orit Fisher and Ruth Traub Bar-Ilan*

School of Occupational Therapy, Hadassah and Hebrew University,
Mount Scopus, Jerusalem

ABSTRACT

This chapter will describe an integrative cognitive functional intervention designed to complement pharmacological treatment for children with ADHD. The intervention is theoretically grounded in the World Health Organization model of health implications, the International Classification of Functioning Disability and Health (ICF) (WHO 2001) which explains the bio-psycho-social factors that impede participation and quality of life. The Cog-Fun is an applied cognitive rehabilitation model, which addresses neurocognitive and psycho-social challenges in a real world context. In this chapter we will present this theoretical understanding of ADHD implications, the proposed change mechanisms of the Cog-Fun and research evidence in children with ADHD.

INTRODUCTION

Attention deficit hyperactivity disorder (ADHD) is a childhood-onset disorder that is considered one of the most common neurobehavioral disorders and among the most prevalent chronic health conditions (American Academy of Pediatrics, 2011). It is an early-onset and enduring disorder, characterized by developmental deficits in attention, increased hyperactivity and impulsivity, resulting in impairments in multiple domains of personal life

---

[*] Correspondence: Adina Maeir, Ph.D. School of Occupational Therapy, Hadassah and Hebrew University PO Box 24026, Mount Scopus, Jerusalem, 91240, E-mail: adina.maeir@huji.mail.ac.il.

(American Psychiatric Association, 2013). The prevalence of ADHD among children and adolescence is estimated to range between 3.7%-8.9% of all children worldwide (Polanczyk, deLima, Horta, Biederman, & Rohde, 2007). ADHD has been shown to profoundly disrupt functioning throughout the life cycle, to increase the risk for educational failure, substance abuse and delinquency (Barkley, Fischer, Smallish, & Fletcher, 2006; Elkins, McGue, & Iacono, 2007; Frazier, Youngstrom, Glutting, & Watkins, 2007; Sibley, et al., 2011). ADHD creates significant barriers to successful participation in a myriad of daily occupations, including play, learning, self-care and social interactions. ADHD has been shown to persist with long-term implications for productivity, family relations, driving, and instrumental activities of daily living, significantly compromising quality of life. (Cermak, & Maeir, 2011).

The extensive ramifications of ADHD are better understood within a broad health perspective which considers both the disorder and its bio-psycho-social consequences. Ustun (2007) suggests that the Family of International Classifications (FIC) of the World Health Organization (WHO, 2001; http://www.who.int/classifications/en/) be applied to the understanding and management of ADHD. The International Classification of Functioning Disability and Health (ICF) complements the International Classification of Diseases (ICD) by describing how health conditions impact body functions and structures, limit activities and restrict participation in life roles. The ICF analyzes health-related functioning in terms of (1) body functions and body structures, (2) activities and participation of the person in society, and (3) contextual factors such as environmental factors and personal factors. The separation of signs/symptoms and consequences permits a better understanding of the disease pathophysiology on the one hand and the consequences on the other hand (Ustun, 2007). In terms of ADHD, the model provides a comprehensive understanding of the impact of ADHD by addressing functional outcomes (activity and participation limitations) as they interact with the biologically derived neurocognitive impairments (body structures and body functions) within the psycho-social context of the individual. The understanding of the complex bio-psycho-social mechanisms that impact the wellbeing of children with ADHD guides the current trends in comprehensive health care for this population (National Institute of Mental Health and Clinical Excellence, 2009; AAP, 2011). The following is a brief account of these mechanisms that form the rationale for the cognitive functional (Cog-Fun) occupational therapy (OT) intervention for children with ADHD (Maeir, Hahn-Markowitz, Fisher, & Traub Bar-Ilan, 2012).

BIO-PSYCHO-SOCIAL IMPLICATIONS OF ADHD

The neurobiological basis of ADHD is well established and the disorder is increasingly recognized as a developmental neurocognitive impairment that involves deficient executive functions (Barkley, 2006; Brown, 2009; Brown, 2013; Willcut, Doyle, Nigg, Faraone, & Pennington, 2005). Executive functions (EF) are higher order cognitive mechanisms responsible for the regulation of cognition, emotion and behavior (Roth, Isquith, & Gioia, 2005). Barkley (2012), defines EF as "those self-directed actions needed to choose goals and to create, enact, and sustain actions towards those goals or more simply as self-regulation to achieve those goals" (p.60). Barkley's theory of EF impairment in ADHD identifies poor inhibition as the core EF deficit which impacts the other EF of working memory, emotional and motivational regulation, internalization of speech, and reconstitution (Barkley, 2006). More recently, Barkley (2012) expanded his theory of EF which now includes self-directed attention – self-awareness which he views as a precursor to all other EF's. This component of self-regulation enables the individual to become aware of their internal and external states, their motivations and actions and so achieves an integrated sense of self which is essential for other self-directed EF. Brown (2009; 2013) also views the EF as the central mechanism of ADHD and delineates six non-hierarchical clusters of EF that tend to be chronically compromised in individuals with ADHD: activation, focus, effort, emotion, memory and action. These functions serve to control and regulate cognition, emotion and behavior to effectively guide one's actions towards future self-serving goals and occupational functioning, particularly in the more complex and dynamic activities of daily living. There is strong evidence supporting the high prevalence of executive dysfunction in ADHD which bears a negative impact on widespread functional outcomes, beyond symptomatology ratings (Stern, Pollack, Bonne, & Maeir, 2013; Willcut, et al., 2005). Therefore, impaired EF have been identified as important targets for intervention in the ADHD population (Cermak & Maeir, 2011). Table 1 illustrates the impact of EF deficits on the occupational domains of children with ADHD.

Table 1. Examples of executive function deficits in occupational domains

Occupation /EF	Play/leisure activities	Activities of Daily living	Learning activities	Social Participation
Inhibition	Doesn't wait his turn, nor play according to rules	Messy eating, doesn't use utensils, leaves table	Answers question (orally or in writing) before he has the entire question	Interrupts friends Talks too much
Effort Recruitment and Persistence	Withdraws from play activities when encountering difficulty	Gives up on being independent in challenging ADLs	Does not finish schoolwork when encounters difficulty	Avoids challenging social situations
Monitoring	Skips steps of activities, omits details	Loses personal belongings	Doesn't check work before submitting assignments	Doesn't check for social cues
Planning and organization	Doesn't consider necessary resources for game in advance (time, equipment)	Disorganized space (messy room), objects (backpack) and action sequence in time (dressing)	Doesn't have the necessary school supplies/books/ assignments	Misses out on social engagements

In addition to deficits in higher level cognitive functioning, it has been shown that the psycho-social context of many individuals with ADHD is also affected. Wehmeir, Schacht & Barkley (2010), explain that the emotional well-being of individuals with ADHD can be compromised due to three distinct factors: (a) the problems inherent in the disorder (e.g., executive-based emotional dysregulation), (b) those related to comorbidity (e.g., ODD, depression, anxiety), and (c) secondary emotional consequences arising from the interaction of ADHD and comorbid disorders with the social environment. These secondary emotional consequences need to be understood within the social and occupational context of the individual. For example, children with ADHD may display a diminished sense of effectiveness due to the difficulties they experience in their daily occupations. This is seen in a reduced degree of enjoyment in and satisfaction from activities that their peers typically engage in and poses a risk for further reduction in participation (Cordier, Bundy, Hocking, & Einfeld, 2010; Dunn, Coster, Cohn, & Orsmond, 2009; Gol & Jarus, 2005). Furthermore, this diminished self-efficacy has also been shown in decreased hope among children with ADHD (Margalit, & Idan, 2004). Hope reflects the individual's belief in his or her ability to find efficient ways to reach desired goals. It enables children to set valued goals, to see the means to achieve those goals, and to find the drive to make those goals happen (Snyder, 2002). Hope is an important personal factor in the management of health challenges as it has been shown to lead to positive adaptation in chronic health conditions among children (Snyder, et al., 1997). The damaged hope found in children with ADHD can be viewed as another example which results from the adverse interaction of core executive deficits with the child's social and occupational context. These secondary emotional impairments further exacerbate the negative functional impact of the disorder.

The family context of the child with ADHD is a critical factor in understanding the functional outcomes and well- being of individuals with ADHD. The literature documents a troubled family setting whereby the family as a system is often trapped in a negative interpersonal cycle, characterized with high levels of stress and difficulties in coping with daily demands (Cussen, Sciberras, Ukoumunne, & Efron, 2012; Davis, Lawrence, Palinkas, Wong, & Leslie, 2011; McIntyre, & Hennessy, 2012). Studies of parent's experiences with raising a child with ADHD reveal the caring responsibility as overwhelming (Peters, & Jackson, 2009). The daily challenges leave parents exhausted physically and emotionally. There is an ongoing mismatch between parental expectations, intentions and effort with outcomes. They perceive ongoing failure in their parenting which leads to frustration, reduced parental efficacy, anxiety, guilt and shame. The perception of their children is often fragmented and colored by their negative daily struggles which overlook their children's strengths. This negative perception is often exacerbated by poor understanding of the source of their child's difficulties and misattribution of their problems to non-biological factors (Moldavsky, & Sayal, 2013). Considering this body of evidence it is imperative that the family context be addressed in any effective treatment process for improving the current and future functioning of the child with ADHD (Whalen, Odgers, Reed, & Henker, 2011).

In summary, the literature supports the involvement of bio-psycho-social mechanisms that influence the outcomes of individuals with ADHD. Existing pharmacological and psychosocial interventions have been shown to be effective in improving ADHD symptomatology and behavioral outcomes of children (AAP, 2011). However, there is a need for family–centered and occupation based interventions that address core executive dysfunction in a broader psychosocial and occupational context.

THE COG-FUN MODEL

The Cog-Fun integrative practice model was designed to target the neurocognitive, emotional and environmental barriers as they interact in occupational contexts. The Cog-Fun is grounded in an occupational therapy (OT) paradigm, in line with the ICF, that considers occupation and participation in life roles as a central determinant of health and well–being (Roley, et al., 2008). The OT paradigm provides a comprehensive understanding of interactions among Person, Environment and Occupation (PEO) factors in order to explain the complexity of occupational performance. Thus, holistic cognitive rehabilitation models in OT, address the neurocognitive health challenges of their clients from this PEO perspective. The Cog-Fun is based on the assumption that there are multiple pathways involved in successful adaptation to ADHD that involve PEO factors. Therefore, the essential neurocognitive deficit of children with ADHD is viewed in the broader PEO (bio-psycho-social) context of their lives. Accordingly, positive outcomes for individuals with ADHD have been associated with PEO factors, such as a warm family context, self-awareness, self-efficacy and hope, efficient strategy use and a good person-occupation fit (Brooks, 2002; Cermak, & Maeir 2011). The objectives of the Cog-Fun are to improve participation in daily occupations, promote executive strategy acquisition and emergent awareness, improve occupational self–efficacy, empower and enable parents as mediators of the above, and finally to improve quality of life of the child and family. These objectives are achieved through the integrative implementation of treatment principles and methods originating from established OT conceptual models. This integrative approach was designed to harness multiple change mechanisms in order to enable successful adaptation to ADHD (see figure 1). The primary therapeutic objective of the Cog-Fun is to promote the acquisition of executive strategies and self-efficacy in occupational performance. The strategies were designed to effectively compensate for the neurocognitive EF barriers to participation. In order for these strategies to be internalized they need to part of the child's occupational context and "language", acquired in enjoyable and fun activities, and to be experienced as tools that are worth the effort. The effortful strategy learning is imparted within a positive, family-centered therapeutic setting and with environmental supports. This integrative approach employs three key change mechanisms.

The first change mechanism is executive strategy acquisition, a metacognitive learning process that is designed to bypass or overcome the cognitive deficits in occupational performance. The integration of metacognitive learning with occupational performance is portrayed in the Multi -Context Treatment Approach (MTA) in cognitive rehabilitation (Toglia, 2011). The MTA targets processing strategies and self-awareness which are considered modifiable constructs within the person, especially the person with mild to moderate neurological involvement. The hypothesized underlying mechanisms of change are awareness and strategy competence, relying on language and declarative learning that facilitate top-down controlled behavior in multiple contexts. Core elements of the MTA include strategy self-generation and explicit transfer training; enhancing self-monitoring and self-awareness; use of everyday activities that are tailored to the client's level and interests. These elements are hypothesized to enhance the probability of transfer of learning to diverse occupational domains. In the Cog-Fun the EF strategy acquisition is broken down into several steps. At first the child experiences the need and advantages of using an executive strategy in a variety of activities (e.g., the need for inhibition - "Stop" strategy, is experienced in running and stopping in the game "red light green light"; or the need for recruiting effort is experienced in a "tug of war" game or pushing against a large ball). The child then names the strategy, and creates a tangible symbol of the strategy (e.g., stop sign sticker, the word "stop", or 'Mr. Effort, "the Force" or an action figure from the child's play-world) that is transferred to multiple activities and contexts in therapy and at home. These executive strategies are practiced with the child and parent and transferred to occupational goals. The playful activities and goals are selected with child and parent and designed to harness motivational and cognitive resources towards goal-oriented behavior. The metacognitive learning process also involves a gradual development of self-awareness, incorporating both online and intellectual awareness (Toglia, & Kirk, 2000). Online awareness is facilitated through the guided acquisition of EF strategies where the child learns to recognize when a strategy is needed during activity engagement. The structured therapeutic activities provide the cognitive supports to enable the discovery of EF challenges. Once the child has a tool (e.g., 'stop' strategy) to cope with an EF deficit (e.g., impulsivity) he is more able to monitor his actions and reflect on them, thus supporting intellectual awareness. In addition, the empowerment that the child experiences by using strategies to improve his performance, helps him realize that the lack of control (e.g., impulsivity) in his actions does not serve his purposes and that he has an effective alternative. Thus, the experience of occupational strategy efficacy reduces the psychogenic threat in acknowledging deficits and promotes adaptive self-awareness. Adaptive self-awareness is defined as a balanced awareness of strengths, challenges and strategies that support occupational performance (as opposed to maladaptive awareness which impedes occupational performance). Metacognitive learning is a highly effective adaptive mechanism for individuals with mild to moderate cognitive deficits, yet it is an effortful, time consuming and gradual process. Therefore, it is necessary to supplement this learning with other adaptive techniques in order to boost motivation and also meet the immediate family needs for daily functioning.

The second change mechanism is procedural learning and environmental supports based on the Neurofunctional Training (NFT) approach to cognitive rehabilitation (Guiles, 2011). The NFT utilizes behavioral learning and environmental resources, confining the need for higher level cognitive process and minimizing frustration during the learning process. One component of NFT is task specific behavioral learning which focuses on achieving specific functional goals. The targeted functional task is broken down to small chunks, probability of errors largely reduced, behaviors practiced, reinforced and 'over-learned'. As opposed to metacognitive treatment, task specific learning is designed to minimize effort and enable relatively rapid success in designated tasks that are of high motivational significance to the client. Learning is task specific and there is no expectation of transfer to other tasks, yet an improvement in self-efficacy and other volitional factors is often found. The underlying change mechanisms are implicit procedural learning processes which bypass the executive deficit area. The other component of NFT is environmental supports and adaptations. Environmental adaptations for individuals with cognitive disabilities concentrate on enabling function and participation through modifying factors that are external to the individual. The physical and human factors in the clients' environment are adapted to the cognitive profile of the individual based on theories of cognitive task analysis and understanding of the person-environment interface. The hypothesized mechanism of change is the suitability of the adaptation (environment-person fit) and the impact of environmental factors on health and well-being. Adaptations depend on the presence and availability of environmental resources. The Cog-Fun implements these methods by creating a well-defined structure to the treatment sessions, adapting activities to the child's level and providing cues, which together reduce the EF demands and enable successful performance. These techniques are modeled for the parents who are guided and encouraged to provide the suitable adaptations for their child in their natural environments outside the clinic. Both task specific training and environmental adaptations are implemented in the Cog-Fun to boost motivation and self-efficacy within a relatively short time period, in order to supplement the more effortful metacognitive learning when necessary.

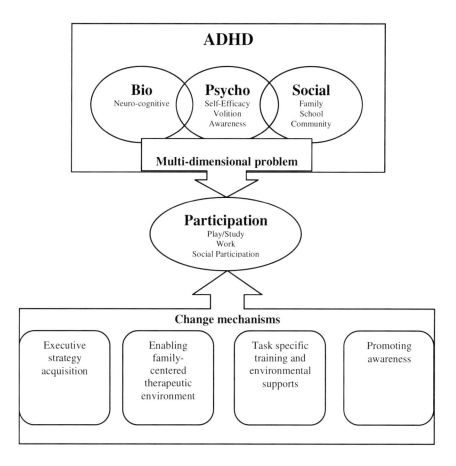

Figure 1. The implications of ADHD and proposed change mechanisms.

The third change mechanism is the enabling therapeutic setting. The setting is child-centered, family-centered and focused on the unique motivations of each client. The positive, warm, safe setting is designed to promote an enabling social context for the children, both in therapy and at home. This enabling social context is achieved through a focus on the volition of the child and parents, as guided by the Model of Human Occupation (MOHO) (Kielhofner, 2008). The MOHO model provides a theoretical understanding of the factors that enable occupational performance and explains how occupation is motivated (Volition system), patterned (Habituation system), and performed (Performance system). The Cog-Fun draws on the MOHO conceptualization of the volition system, comprising values, interests and personal causation, as a key factor in targeting the psychological implications of ADHD. Seeking out and strengthening the child's motivations for occupation is central for creating a sound and healing foundation for the prolonged journey with ADHD. Furthermore, the enabling social context created in the Cog-Fun intervention is achieved through therapeutic use of self, interpersonal reasoning, therapeutic communication and family centeredness, derived from the Intentional Relationship Model (IRM) (Taylor, 2008). The IRM delineates six therapeutic communication modes: (empathy, encouraging, empathizing, collaborating, problem solving, instructing and advocating) that are used in an intentional and flexible manner. This intentional relationship is essential for addressing the complex learning challenges faced by the child (e.g., learning EF strategies) and the parent (e.g., reframing their child's challenges in a neurobiological health perspective and understanding their role in providing appropriate supports to enable optimal functioning). Both the MOHO and the IRM provide the tools to address the impaired psycho-social context that is jeopardized by ADHD.

In summary, the Cog-Fun is a psycho-social treatment model designed to complement pharmacotherapy for ADHD, integrating multiple change mechanisms to facilitate a positive adaptation process for the child with ADHD.

THE COG-FUN PROTOCOL

The Cog-Fun is a manualized treatment approach (Maeir, et al., 2012) administered by licensed OT's that receive certification from a Cog-Fun training course. A unique facet of the intervention is the combination of structure with flexibility. The structure provides the necessary clarity and supports to enable effective learning for families with ADHD, while the flexibility considers the unique individual profile of each client. The treatment principles are described in Table 2. The treatment format comprises a weekly one hour treatment session with child and parent over 13-14 weeks. The protocol comprises seven intervention units: evaluation, four units of executive strategy acquisition (addressing inhibition, effort, monitoring and planning), home visit and summary unit. The strategy units are designed in a developmental hierarchy and focus first on the basic EF strategies ('stop' , 'recruit effort') and then on the more advanced strategies ('check', 'plan'). The guidelines are to teach one strategy at a time and proceed according to the client's progress. Therefore, not all strategies will be imparted to every client. A more detailed description of the intervention units is provided in the following case study.

Table 2. Cog-Fun treatment principles

Executive strategy acquisition	
	Provide playful experience demonstrating the need for target strategy
	Create symbolic representation (verbal, visual) for the strategy with the child
	Role reversal to enhance learning, child teaches strategy to therapist/parent
	Practice transfer of strategy to multiple activities and link strategy use to individualized occupational goal
	Provide explicit and specific reinforcement of strategy use (regardless of outcome)
	Verify that strategies are used in activities with the "just right challenge" for the child to enable experiencing the value of the strategy.
	Maintain strategy motivation (be cautious of overusing strategies)
	Parent training in strategy acquisition and transfer

Enabling setting	
	Flexible use of therapeutic modes
	Active attention to and discovery of clients' (child and parent) strengths, interests and motivating factors
	Maintaining playful, fun and emotionally safe environment
	Empowering clients through choice, active engagement and role reversal
	Parents are actively included in treatment activities to the extent that they feel comfortable
	Parent training in creating enabling environment in their home
Environmental supports and task specific learning	
	Treatment sessions are supported with a structured routine including introducing activities on activity board, use of timer, checking activities and notebook summary
	Adapting task/environment to enable success (preparing parts of activity in advance, removing distractors, etc)
	Use of regulating activities when needed (squeezing ball, jumping on one foot, etc,) in order to proceed with treatment agenda
	Task specific training for designated occupations with high significance for child or parent (getting dressed, tying shoes, etc)
	Parent training in using EF supports in their environments
Occupational goal setting	
	Occupational goal setting is a process that begins in the evaluation and continues throughout the intervention
	Goals are occupation - based, defined in specific, measurable, attainable and positive terms
	Executive strategies are embedded in goal definitions when possible (e.g., will 'check' his backpack before going to sleep)
	Parent training in occupational goal setting
Promoting awareness	
	Evaluate parents' knowledge and attitudes towards ADHD in advance, referral to information sources and discussion
	Provide time and support for explicit reflection on EF challenges/strengths in activity performance
	Always ensure that awareness promotion occurs in a context of strengths and strategy skills to prevent psychogenic resistance
	Parent training to foster adaptive awareness

CASE STUDY

David is a 6 year old boy with ADHD (Hyperactive -Impulsive) that received the Cog-Fun intervention. The following describes the intervention units which took place over 13 sessions in the Cog-Fun lab.

Unit I –Evaluation and Introduction of Cog-Fun

The first evaluation meeting was conducted with the parents. The interview focused on David's developmental history, executive functioning - using the Behavior Rating Inventory of Executive Functions (BRIEF) (Gioia, Isquith, Guy, & Kenworthy, 2000), occupational profile (ADL, play, learning, leisure, and social participation), family resources and preferences. In addition, we discussed the issue of David's ADHD diagnosis, evaluating their knowledge and attitudes towards the diagnosis as well as how they talk about ADHD with their son. We introduced the Cog-Fun principles and the central role they will have as parents in the intervention process. The results of the parent interview revealed their perception of

David as a bright and a creative boy whose strengths are overshadowed by marked impulsivity that interferes with the quality of his performance in many occupations. They described the challenges during mealtimes when he leaves the table quickly, spills beverages and food, doesn't finish his meals (they were worried about his low weight), and during playtime when he bullies his younger brother. They were also concerned about his limited social participation with friends and his difficulties in school (kindergarten). They seemed helpless in the face of ongoing complaints from his teacher regarding his disruptive behavior in school. It appeared that the parents did not know a lot about the diagnosis of ADHD except for the pharmacological treatment which was currently ruled out for medical reasons. Since David was their oldest son they didn't know what to expect. They just knew that despite his intelligence and charm, the day- to- day routine had become frustrating for everyone in the family. Although they were expecting another child they said that they were willing to commit to the program and mentioned the availability of additional help from their own parents. Following assessment, using the Canadian Occupational Performance Measure (COPM) (Law, et al., 2005) we set goals together with the parents: Goal 1 'David will stop before hitting his 3 year old brother and hit a pillow instead'. Goal 2 'during circle time (in school), David will succeed to stop before interrupting / hitting / disrupting and tell the teacher when he needs a break'; Goal 3 'David will recruit effort and call a friend on the phone and invite him over'; and Goal 4 'at dinner time, David will recruit effort, set a timer for 10 minutes and sit with the family'.

The next session focused on establishing the therapeutic alliance with David, who was informed by his parents to bring a game from home. The session began with introducing the therapist and the room saying that we will meet every week, play and learn new things. David was asked about the things he likes to do, with whom and etc. He was asked if he knows why he came to O.T. treatment. We continued with the assessment of David's EF challenges by using the Pictorial Interview of Children's Meta-cognition & Executive functions (PIC-ME) (Traub Bar-Ilan, et al., 2013). The PICME includes 34 scenarios depicting executive challenges in the daily lives of children. The client rates the frequency which he encounters similar difficulties and the extent to which it bothers him. The PICME is used to assess the child's awareness of his EF difficulties and also to set client-centered goals. Following the PIC-ME we played two games, one in which David chose from a given repertoire, and the other was the game he had brought from home. While playing with David we observed his cognitive and social interaction skills. The assessment and observation presented a bright, sensitive child, very fun and engaging in play, yet with marked impulsivity and restlessness. He showed lack of awareness to most of his EF difficulties, although he did recognize himself in three items of the PICME portraying a child that gets extremely upset when someone annoys him (item 20); that does some things without thinking and then regrets them (item 29); that has difficulty keeping clean and tidy (item 36). David rated himself as often having difficulties on these items, that they disturbed him and that he would like to change them. In this session he was also introduced to some of the Cog-Fun routines and resources, the 'Activity chart' that is used to plan every session, the timer and "my Cog-Fun notebook" to summarize the session.

Units II-III Strategy Acquisition: Inhibit, Effort

Over the next six sessions David was introduced to his 'new friends', the executive strategies represented by graphic symbols and pictures: 'Mr. Stop' and 'Mr. Effort'. At first, David was exposed to the challenge of stopping during playful activities. He gained more credits as he improved in stopping, for example, stopping before picking up a wrong card; stopping his body responses in conflicting situations (e.g., "Simon says"). Strategy acquisition required modeling the use of stop, and a lot of reinforcement to any expression of controlled behavior.

The effort strategy (Mr. Effort) was similarly introduced to further sustain controlled behavior over time. Both parents were involved in therapy (one of them in each session) and took part in a playful, fun, safe atmosphere that offered the "just right challenge". They both took a major part in mediating the strategies to David. The mother, who was very critical of David at the beginning, started seeing his playfulness and the emergence of his more controlled behavior. She then joined the activities and began to mediate the use and application of 'stop' strategies. The parents borrowed games, printed and played with the strategy symbols and practiced this playful work at home. Between sessions they documented their successes and challenges and maintained communication with therapists by email. When we felt that David's self - efficacy was growing along with his parent's confidence in using EF language, we started to work on their occupational goals involving the need to stop and recruit effort. Prior to coping with the 'real life' challenge of stopping before hitting his brother, we practiced this challenge in a safe environment, using role playing and simulated tasks. At this point the parents suggested including the kindergarten teacher in the process. David and his parents introduced her to the Cog-Fun symbols and the teacher suggested that David teach them to his classmates. She also offered that at circle time David will sit next to her (adaptation). David also used an internal script (internalization of strategies) "When I feel angry or restless (my heart beats fast, I want to cry / hit / shout) I raise my hand as a 'stop' sign or touch the teacher. I stop and recruit effort till the teacher signals to me that I can leave the room". The units (IV and V) for acquisition of more advanced EF strategies (check and plan) were not introduced at this stage, since we evaluated that David had not yet fully mastered the prerequisite basic strategies.

Unit VI – Home Visit

The home visit is an important feature of the transfer-of-learning process. David was very excited about the visit which gave him an opportunity to demonstrate what he had acquired during the treatment process. He took charge of the visit and prepared for it in advance with his mother. David demonstrated how he set the timer during mealtime and succeeded to sit for 10 minutes during mealtime. He then played with us a game of his choice and invited his brother to join us. During the game, the therapist asked David to help her use the EF strategies when she role-played dysregulated behavior.

Unit VII – Summary and Wrap-Up

Finally, unit 7 included two sessions which focused on preparing David towards completing the intervention. We planned the last session in advance through role play and using the activity chart to determine the activities we would like to do and the strategies we will need to use. Following the activity a creative project of his choice was used to summarize the Cog-Fun intervention. The treatment conclusion with parents involved discovering what they had learned from the Cog-Fun experience. Parents' ratings after treatment demonstrated clinically significant improvement on the behavioral regulation scales of the BRIEF and the COPM. Furthermore, they expressed better understanding of David's ADHD and his EF's challenges and more confidence in managing their daily challenges. They felt more competent in setting realistic goals, supporting strategy acquisition, adapting their environment and seeking support as needed. They further expressed satisfaction from David's acquired strategies which were reflected mainly in increased self- control in his social participation. "David believes that he is capable of using strategies to achieve goals that are important to him at home and at kindergarten. They were also very pleased with the dramatic change in the teacher's attitude towards David.

RESEARCH

The Cog-Fun proposes that an integrative cognitive approach to children with ADHD will improve daily functioning in the present and set the foundations in the child and his environment to promote participation in life roles in the future. It is assumed that clients who enter these positive pathways at an earlier stage in life will have more opportunities for achieving better functional outcomes than those depicted in the outcome literature on ADHD. Initial supporting evidence for the effectiveness of the Cog-Fun has been demonstrated in two studies among children ages 5-9 years old (Hahn–Markowitz, Manor, & Maeir, 2011; Maeir, Fisher, Traub Bar-Ilan, Boas, Berger & Landau, 2014). The first pilot study (N=17), utilized a one sample, pre-post design and demonstrated significant moderate to large effects of Cog-Fun treatment in children ages 7-9 (see Table 3). A significant treatment effect was found for the main outcome measures, the COPM and the BRIEF. Moreover, the post-intervention effect was maintained at 3-months follow-up. In addition, significant effects were found for measures of self-efficacy (children's COPM) and neuropsychological measure of attention, the Test of Variables of Attention (TOVA; Greenberg, et al., 1996), planning, the Tower of London (TOL; Culbertson, & Zillmer, 2005) and organization, the Rey Osterrieth Complex Figure (ROCF; Osterrieth, 1944). Furthermore, parent ratings showed significant reduction in symptoms of ADHD, on the Conner's Rating Scales-Revised (CPRS-R, Conner, 2000) and improved quality of life, on the Pediatric Quality of Life 4.0 Generic Core Scales (PedsQL, parent version; Varni, & Burwinkle, 2006). A second study (Maeir, et al., 2014) utilized a controlled crossover design (N=19) with two groups (research group and waitlist controls) of children aged 5-7 years old. Significant moderate to large treatment effects on both the COPM and BRIEF were found after treatment. Comparison between research and controls revealed significant group X time interaction effects on the BRIEF and COPM, with improved occupational and EF outcomes for the research group and a trend to worsening outcomes in the waitlist controls. The positive treatment effects were replicated in the control group after crossover to treatment and gains were maintained in both groups at three months follow-up. The findings of these two studies provide initial support for the efficacy of Cog-Fun intervention for improving executive functioning and participation in children with ADHD. A randomized controlled trial is currently underway with 100 children from two central ADHD cites in Israel.

Table 3. Cog-Fun pilot intervention results

Measures	Pre M (SD)	Post M (SD)	Effect Size Hedge's *g*	FU M (SD)
Occupational Performance:				
COPM Parent	3.71 (1.57)	7.81 (1.03)**	3.00	7.04 (1.21)
Executive Functions:				
1 BRIEF P GEC (T)	67.14 (8.87)	58.57 (12.05)**	.79	59.33 (12.03)
2 BRIEF T GEC (T)	57.82 (8.13)	52.10 (6.70) **	.74	54.20 (6.99)
3 ToL Total Moves (SS)	89.38 (18.41)	106.00 (13.74)*	1.00	99.38 (13.55)
4 ToL Total Rule Violations (SS)	83.85 (18.86)	95.85 (17.14)*	.65	92.62 (20.12)
5 ROCF Copy Total Score	18.46 (8.47)	21.23 (9.03)*	.31	21.55 (8.85)
6 ROCF Organizational Score	4.00 (.913)	4.31 (.855)*	.34	4.36 (1.12)
Quality of Life:				
PedsQoL P Psychosocial Mean	59.41 (11.96)	67.74 (17.77)*	.53	66.81 (15.28)
ADHD symptoms:				
CPS-R (T) ADHD Index	70.43 (10.22)	63.50 (10.68)*	.64	65.17 (9.10)
CTS-R (T) ADHD Index	57.10 (10.13)	53.70 (7.26)	.37	55.90 (8.75)
Self-efficacy: COPM Child				
Performance of Goals	3.77 (1.86)	8.46 (3.36)**	1.68	7.78 (2.02)
Attention: TOVA* **				
Omission Total SS	63.08 (27.816)		.56	78.08 (24.216)*
Commission Total SS	99.62 (13.506)		.21	102.92 (16.864)

* < .05.
** < .01.
*** The TOVA was administered prior to intervention and at follow-up.
SD=Standard Deviation, FU=Follow-Up, C=Child, P=Parents, COPM=Canadian Occupational Performance Measure, BRIEF=Behavior Rating Inventory of Executive Functions, GEC=Global Executive Composite, T=T score, ToL=Tower of London, SS=Standard Score, ROCF=Rey Osterreich Complex Figure, Org'al=Organizational, PedsQoL=Pediatric Quality of Life Generic Scales, CPS-R/CTS-R=Conner's Parent/Teacher Scales-Revised, TOVA=Test of Variables of Attention

In addition to the efficacy studies, the PICME (Traub Bar-Ilan, et al., 2013) evaluation was developed in order to support the Cog-Fun client-centered approach with children. The PICME includes 34 scenarios depicting executive challenges and 10 scenarios depicting areas of strength (such as creativity, kindness and humor) often seen in children with ADHD in their daily lives. The PICME items of EF challenges were shown to have high internal consistency (Cronbach alpha = .96), and responsiveness to treatment (p= .01) regarding items that were identified by the children that they wanted to change (Barami, 2014).

CONCLUSION

This chapter presented the Cog-Fun treatment model which targets the occupational challenges of children with ADHD. The model is an applied cognitive rehabilitation model, which addresses neurocognitive and psycho-social challenges in context. The research evidence provides initial support for the efficacy of the Cog-Fun to improve EF and participation in children with ADHD. We hypothesize that the positive outcomes are likely attributed to a synergistic effect of the learning processes occurring in the child and parents that establish an executive toolbox within a favorable motivational context. Additional research is underway to further examine the efficacy of the Cog-Fun and its' underlying change mechanisms.

REFERENCES

American Academy of Pediatrics. (2011). ADHD: Clinical practice guidelines for the diagnosis, evaluation, and treatment of attention-deficit/ hyperactivity disorder in children and adolescents. *Pediatrics, 128*, 5, 1-16.

American Psychiatric Association (APA), (2013). *DSM-V: Diagnostic and statistical manual of mental disorders* (5th ed.). Washington DC: Author.

Barami, G. (2014). *Responsiveness of the Pictorial Interview of Children's Meta-cognition and Executive functions (PICME) in self-report of children with ADHD and their parents in relation to participation in Cognitive Functional (Cog-Fun) occupational therapy intervention*. MSc. Thesis. Jerusalem: Hebrew University.

Barkley, R. A. (2006). Attention- deficit hyperactivity disorder: A handbook for diagnosis and treatment (3rd ed.). New York, NY: Guilford Press.

Barkley, R. A. (2012). *Executive functions: What they are, how they work, and why they evolved*. New York, NY: Guilford.

Barkley, R. A., Fischer, M., Smallish, L., & Fletcher, K. (2006). Young Adult Outcome of Hyperactive Children: Adaptive Functioning in Major Life Activities. *Journal of American Academy of Child and Adolescents Psychiatry, 45*, 192-202.

Brooks, R. B(2002).Changing the mindset of adults with ADHD: Strategies for fostering hope, optimism, and resilience. In :Goldstein, S. Ellison, A. T. (Eds), (2002). *Clinicians' guide to adult ADHD: Assessment and intervention*. (pp. 127-146). San Diego, CA, US: Academic Press

Brown, T. A. (2013). *New Understanding of ADHD in Children and Adults: Executive Function Impairments*. Routledge, Taylor & Francis Group, NY.

Brown, T. E. (2009). ADD/ADHD and impaired executive function in clinical practice. *Current Attention Disorder Reports*, 1, 37-41.

Cermak, S. A., & Maeir, A. (2011). Cognitive rehabilitation of children and adults with attention- deficit/ hyperactivity disorder. In N. Katz (Ed.), *Cognition, Occupation and*

Participation across the Life Span (pp. 249-276). American Occupational Therapy Association, Inc. MD: Bethesda.

Conner, K. C. (2000). *Conners' Rating Scales-Revised*. North Tonawanda, NY: Multi-Health Systems Inc.

Cordier, R., Bundy, A., Hocking, C., & Einfeld, S. (2010). Empathy in the Play of Children with Attention Deficit Hyperactivity Disorder. *OTJR: Occupation, Participation and Health, 30* (3), 122-132.

Cussen, A., Sciberras, E., Ukoumunne, O.C., Efron, D. (2012). Relationship between symptoms of attention-deficit hyperactivity disorder and family functioning: A community-based study. *European Journal of Pediatrics, 171,* 271–280

Culbertson, W. C., & Zillmer, E. A. (2005). *Tower of London Drexel University: 2nd Edition (TOL^{DX}), Technical Manual*. North Tonawanda, NY: Multi-Health Systems Inc.

Davis, C.C., Lawrence, M.C., Palinkas, A., Wong, J. B. &. Leslie, L.K. (2011). Putting families in the center: Family perspectives on decision making and ADHD and implications for ADHD care. *Journal of Attention Disorders, 16,* 675-684.

Dunn, L., Coster, W., Cohn, E. S., & Orsmond, G. I. (2009). Factors Associated with Participation of Children With and Without ADHD in Household Tasks. *Physical and Occupational Therapy in Pediatrics, 29*(3), 274-294.

Elkins, I. J., McGue, M., &Iacono, W. G. (2007). Prospective effects of attention-deficit/hyperactivity disorder, conduct disorder, and sex on adolescent substance use and abuse. *Archives of General Psychiatry, 64,* 1145-1152.

Frazier, T. W., Youngstrom, E. A., Glutting, J. J, & Watkins, M. W. (2007).ADHD and achievement: meta-analysis of the child, adolescent, and adult literatures and a concomitant study with college students. *Journal of Learning Disabilities, 40,* 49-65.

Gol, D., & Jarus, T. (2005). Effect of a social skills training group on everyday activities of children with attention-deficit-hyperactivity disorder. *Developmental Medicine & Child Neurology, 47,* 539-545.

Gioia, G. A., Isquith, P. K., Guy, S. C., & Kenworthy, L. (2000). *Behavior Rating Inventory of Executive Function (BRIEF)*. Odessa, FL: Psychological Assessment Resources.

Greenberg, L., Leark, R. A., Dupy, T. R., Corman, C. L., Kindschi, R. N., & Cenedela, M. (1996). *T.O.V.A.: Test of variables of attention: Clinical guide*. Los Alimitos: Universal Attention Disorders.

Guiles, G. M. (2011). A Neurofunctional approach to rehabilitation after brain injury. In N. Katz (Ed.), *Cognition, Occupation and Participation across the Life Span* (pp. 351-382). American Occupational Therapy Association, Inc. MD: Bethesda.

Hahn- Markowitz, J., Manor, I., & Maeir, A. (2011). Effectiveness of cognitive functional (Cog-Fun) intervention with children with attention deficit hyperactivity disorder: A pilot study. *American Journal of Occupational Therapy, 65(4),* 384-392.

Kielhofner, G. (2008). *Model of Human Occupation: Theory and Application* (4th ed.). Baltimore: Lippincott Williams & Wilkins.

Law, M., Baptiste, S., Carswell, A., McColl, M. A., Polatajko, H., & Pollock, N. (2005a). *The Canadian Occupational Performance Measure* (4th ed.). Ottawa, ON: CAOT Publications Ace.

Maeir. A., Hahn- Markowitz, J., Fisher, O. & Traub Bar-Ilan, R. (2012). *Cognitive functional (Cog-Fun) intervention in occupational therapy for children aged 5-10 with ADHD:*

Treatment Manual. Jerusalem: School of Occupational Therapy, Faculty of Medicine, Hadassah and Hebrew University.

Maeir, A. Fisher, O., Traub Bar-Ilan, R., Boas, N., Berger, I. Landau, Y. (2014). Effectiveness of cognitive–functional (Cog–Fun) occupational therapy intervention for young children with Attention Deficit Hyperactivity Disorder: A controlled study. *American Journal of Occupational Therapy, 68(3) 1-8.*

Margalit, M., & Idan, O. (2004). Resilience and Hope Theory: An Expanded Paradigm for Learning Disabilities Research. *Thalamus, 22*(1), 58-64.

McIntyre, R., & Hennessy, H., (2012). 'He's just enthusiastic. Is that such a bad thing?' Experiences of parents of children with Attention Deficit Hyperactivity Disorder. *Emotional and Behavioural Difficulties 17*, 1, 65–82.

Moldavsky, M., & Sayal, K. (2013). Knowledge and Attitudes about Attention-Deficit/Hyperactivity Disorder (ADHD) and its Treatment: The Views of Children, Adolescents, Parents, Teachers and Healthcare Professionals. *Current Psychiatry Reports, 15*(8) 1-7.

National Institute of Mental Health and Clincal Excellence. (2009). *Attention deficit hyperactivity disorder: Diagnosis and management of ADHD in children, young people and adults* (NICE Clinical Guideline No. 72). London, UK: Author.

Osterrieth, P. A. (1944). Le test de copie d'une figure complexe. *Archives Psychology, 30*, 206 -356.

Peters, K. & Jackson, D. (2009) Mothers' experiences of parenting a child with attention deficit hyperactivity disorder. *Journal of Advanced Nursing 65(1),* 62–71

Polanczyk, G., deLima, M. S., Horta, B. L., Biederman, J., & Rohde, A. (2007). The Worldwide Prevalence of ADHD: A Systematic Review Metaregression Analysis. *The American Journal of Psychiatry, 164(6), 942-948.*

Roley, S. S., DeLany, J. V., Barrows, C. J., Brownrigg, S., Honaker, D., Sava, D. I., & Youngstrom, M. J. (2008). Occupational therapy practice framework: domain & practice. *The American journal of Occupational Therapy 62,* (6), 625.

Roth, R. M., Isquith, P. K., & Gioia, G. A. (2005). *Behavior Rating Inventory of Executive Function – Adult version.* Lutz, FL: Psychological Assessment Resources, Inc.

Sibley, M. H., Pelham, W. E., Molina, B. S. G., Gnagy, E. M., Waschbusch, D. A., Biswas, A., Karch, K. (2011). The delinquency outcomes of boys with ADHD with and without comorbidity. *Journal of Abnormal Child Psychology, 39,* 21–32.

Snyder, C. R. (2002). Hope theory: Rainbows in the Mind. *Psychological Inquiry, 13*(4), 249-275.

Snyder, C. R., Hoza, B., Pelham, W. E., Rapoff, M., Ware, L., Danovsky, M., Highberger, L., Rubinstein, H., & Stahl, K. J. (1997). The Development and Validation of the Children's Hope Scale. *Journal of Pediatric Psychology, 22*(3), 399-421.

Stern, A., Pollack, Y., Bonne, O., Malik, E., & Maeir, A. (2013). The relationship between executive functions and quality of life in adults with ADHD. Journal of Attention Disorders. Advance online publication. *http://dx.doi.org/10.1177/1087054713504133.*

Taylor, R. R. (2008). *The Intentional Relationship: Occupational Therapy and the Use of Self.* Philadelphia: F. A. Davis.

Toglia, J. P. (2011). The dynamic interactional model of cognition in cognitive rehabilitation. In N. Katz (Ed.), *Cognition, Occupation and Participation across the Life Span* (pp. 161-202). American Occupational Therapy Association, Inc. MD. `

Toglia, J., & Kirk, U. (2000).Understanding awareness deficits following brain injury. *NeuroRehabilitation, 15,* 57–70.

Traub Bar-Ilan, R., Cohen, N., Amsily Yahbess, O., Dekel, S., Hoori, H., Barami, G., Vaizman-Dill, Z., & Maeir, A (2014). *Pictorial Interview of Children's Meta-cognition & Executive functions (PIC-ME) Test Manual.* Jerusalem: School of Occupational Therapy, Hadassah and Hebrew University.

Ustun, T.B. (2007). Using the international classification of functioning, disease and health in attention-deficit/hyperactivity disorder: separating the disease from its epiphenomena. *Ambulatory Pediatrics*, 7, 132-9.

Varni, J. W., & Burwinkle, T. M. (2006). The PedsQLTM as a patient-reported outcome in children and adolescents with Attention-Deficit/Hyperativity Disorder: A population-based study. *Health and Quality of Life Outcomes, 4*(26), 4-26.

Wehmeier, P. M., Schacht, A., & Barkley, R. A. (2010). Social and emotional impairment in children and adolescents with ADHD and the impact on quality of life. *Journal of Adolescent Health. 46,* 209-217.

Whalen, C. K.; Odgers, C. L.; Reed, P. L.; Henker, B. (2011). Dissecting daily distress in mothers of children with ADHD: An electronic diary study. *Journal of Family Psychology 25*(3), 402-411.

Willcutt, E.G., Doyle, A.E., Nigg, J.T., Faraone, S.V., & Pennington, B.F. (2005).Validity of the executive function theory of attention-deficit/hyperactivity disorder: A meta-analytic review, *Biological Psychiatry, 57,* 1336–1346.

World Health Organization. (2001). *International Classification of Functioning, Disability and Health (ICF).* Geneva: Author.

In: ADHD
Editors: Itai Berger and Adina Maeir

ISBN: 978-1-63321-047-9
© 2014 Nova Science Publishers, Inc.

Chapter 7

ADHD AMONG CHILDREN WITH SIGNIFICANT DEVELOPMENTAL DELAY OR INTELLECTUAL DISABILITY

Michal Begin[*], *M.D.*

Developmental Pediatrician, Leumit HMO, Jerusalem, Israel
Pediatrician, Hadassah Medical Center, Jerusalem, Israel

ABSTRACT

Intellectual disability (ID) involves impairment of general mental abilities that impact adaptive functioning. Symptoms of ADHD have been frequently observed in children with ID and traditionally have been considered by clinicians and researchers to be consistent with the delayed developmental age. In recent years, there is increasing evidence to support the validity in clinical utility of making a diagnosis of ADHD in people with ID. The diagnosis of ADHD allows medical treatment that may alleviate some behavioral symptoms that are distressful to family and teachers. Treatment of ADHD symptoms may minimize the effect of intellectual limitation on adaptive functions and may allow children with ID to fully realize their learning potential in school setting. The following chapter is a brief review of the most common genetic conditions associated with ID and recent data on the prevalence, presentation of symptoms and treatment of ADHD in these syndromes.

INTRODUCTION

Intellectual disability (ID) involves impairment of general mental abilities that impact adaptive functioning. The DSM5 addresses the impact of ID on a person's function and uses 3 domains to describe how well an individual can cope with everyday tasks:

---

[*] Correspondence: Dr. Michal Begin, 3 Trumpeldor St, Jerusalem, Israel, 9459003. E-mail: mbegin@leumit.co.il.

- Conceptual domains (e.g.: language, reading, writing, math etc.)
- Social domains (e.g.: empathy, social judgment, interpersonal communication skills)
- Practical domains (e.g.: personal care, job responsibility, money management, etc.)

Although the DSM5 removed IQ from the criteria they are still used in the description of the intellectual disability and an IQ must be approximately 2 standard deviations or more below the population (IQ score of 70 or below) in addition to assessment of function in the 3 domains.

ID affects approximately 3% of the general population in developed countries (WHO 1992, APA 2000). In a meta-analysis of population based studies the prevalence of ID in the general population was 10.37/ 1000 [1], with the highest rates in countries with low and middle income. While the prevalence of developmental disabilities in general has been on the rise in the US in recent years, the prevalence of intellectual disabilities has dropped 1.5% in the United States [2]. This may be due to changes in accuracy of diagnosis e.g., more children having an early diagnosis of autism or a learning disability.

Symptoms of ADHD have been frequently observed in children with ID and traditionally have been considered by clinicians and researchers to be consistent with the delayed developmental age [3]. Estimates of prevalence of ADHD in population with ID vary from 4% to 42% [4]. Fox [5] reported that 15% of individuals with severe and profound levels of ID may meet diagnostic criteria for ADHD, even when mental age has been taken in the account. Because diagnostic criteria for ADHD emphasize that the symptoms of inattention, hyperactivity and impulsivity must be appropriate for the developmental level, having an ID is in a way discouraging to the clinicians confronting these symptoms because of the difficulty of clearly defining the severity of ADHD symptoms in relation to the degree of ID. Nevertheless, in recent years, there is increasing evidence to support the validity in clinical utility of making a diagnosis of ADHD in people with ID [6, 7, 4]. In fact, identification of ADHD symptoms in children with ID is vital because children with ID and ADHD can have more restrictive school placements, school suspensions, and inpatient psychiatric treatment then children with ID without ADHD [8]. The diagnosis of ADHD allows medical treatment that may alleviate some behavioral symptoms that are distressful to family and teachers. Treatment of ADHD symptoms may minimize the effect of their intellectual limitation on adaptive functions such as improved interpersonal skills and social responsibility, safety, responsible use of money and following routines, and may allow children with ID to fully realize their learning potential in school setting [9].

Intellectual disability is the result of many conditions that effect brain development e.g., perinatal infections, environmental, metabolic, intrauterine exposure and infantile brain trauma. Genetic disorders, as a group, are the major cause of ID in countries where other reasons for ID have diminished (e.g., malnutrition). In this section we will mainly discuss ADHD in children with some of the most common genetic syndromes that may cause intellectual disability: Down syndrome, Fragile X, 22q11.2 deletion and Neurofibromatosis-1.

ADHD IN DOWN SYNDROME

Down syndrome is considered to be the leading major genetic cause of DI. Despite improved prenatal diagnoses, the prevalence of Down syndrome at birth increased from 9.5 to 11.8 per 10,000 births (CDC data 2002). Down syndrome is seen in all ethnic groups. Due to improved medical care children with Down syndrome have a longer life expectancy, and over half of individuals with Down syndrome will live into their 50's [10]. The longer life expectancy introduces issues that are related to adult function such as appropriate schooling that will enhance development of independence [11]. Despite the high prevalence of Down syndrome [12], literature concerning specific learning aspects is scant, and ADHD was mostly studied alongside other psychiatric and neurobehavioral disorders [13,14]. In fact, only one study specifically addressed the question of prevalence of ADHD in Down syndrome, and reported on a prevalence of 43.9% [3]. ADHD diagnosis was not correlated with the degree of intellectual disability in the study group. There was a significant correlation between ADHD symptoms and ophthalmologic problems (mainly refractive errors). The study was not longitudinal and did not report the effect of correction of visual problems on behavior. Despite this flaw, the results of the study emphasize the necessity of regular ophthalmologic evaluation in children and youth with Down syndrome.

Cornish found that children with Down syndrome displayed clinically high levels of inattention symptoms but relatively normal levels of hyperactive symptoms that were comparable to the behavior of younger children matched on their non-verbal mental age [9]. Cornish also reported that in children with Down syndrome who had inattentive behaviors, these were related to poor performance on a variety of measures such as receptive vocabulary, single word reading and letter knowledge, and this was true across time.

MEDICAL TREATMENT OF ADHD IN CHILDREN WITH DOWN SYNDROME

Information on treatment of ADHD symptoms in children with Down syndrome is scant. In a Cochrane review [4] no high level trials of medication for ADHD in Down syndrome (RCTs) were found. In a study published by Ekstein et al. (2011) [3], only 50% of children with Down syndrome who fulfilled criteria for ADHD diagnosis were treated at the time of the study with Methylphenidate. Neither efficacy nor side effects of the medication were discussed in that paper.

ADHD IN FRAGILE X SYNDROME (FXS)

Fragile X Syndrome is considered to be the most common known cause of inherited intellectual disability. The prevalence of FXS is estimated to be 1 in 2500 to 5000 in male and 1 in 4000 to 6000 in female. Fragile X is caused by a mutation of FMR1 gene, located on chromosome Xq27.3. This area is rich with CGG repeats. Up to 54 repeats are considered to be a normal genotype. Individuals with 55 to 199 CGG repeats are considered to have a premutation, and are defined as "carriers" of the mutation. When CGG repeats exceed 200 repeats individuals are considered to have the full mutation. In the full mutation, methylation of the promoter region of the gene occurs, interfering with the production of the fragile X mental retardation protein or FMRP. The neuropathological consequences of decreased FMRP level manifest in the brain as immature dendritic spines and high spine density [15]. FXS patients with the full mutation have cognitive deficits and show distinct behavior features in the areas of attention, hyper arousal, social function, anxiety and aggression [16]. The carrier state is characterized with average cognition, learning disabilities and ADHD and will not be dealt in this chapter because carriers are not considered as having ID.

Animal models with the FMR1 mutant mice recapitulate findings with humans with FXS both in the neuropathological findings [15] and neurobehavioral profile. Mice showed impairments in inhibitory control and attention, and the inhibition deficits became manifest under times of arousal and when confronted with changing task demands [17].

More than 90% of FXS males and 50% females with full mutation meet criteria for ID by school years [15]. The neurocognitive profile in FXS includes difficulties in sequential processing, short term memory deficits, arithmetic problems, attention and inhibitory control problems, fine and gross motor delay and problems with coordination. Because the cognitive growth in children with FXS is approximately half the rate of typically developing children, the intellectual gap between affected and unaffected children widens and there is an age dependent gradual decline in IQ [15].

Initially, symptoms of ADHD were almost synonymous with fragile X syndrome [18]. Currently, ADHD symptoms account for the most prevalent type of problem behavior in FXS documented in the literature [19] and was diagnosed in 54-59% of children bases on a combination of measures in a cohort of 63 children [8]. In a national parent survey, parents of children diagnosed with FXS reported that their child had hyperactivity in 66% of males (30% in females) and reported attention problems in 48% of males (67% in females). High prevalence of related aggression was also reported (38% in males, 14% in females) [20].

Most studies of ADHD symptoms in Fragile X have used parents or teachers report measures. Some researchers have used computerized laboratory tasks to measure visual attention in individuals with FXS, such as the WATT (Wilding Attention Test for Children) and documented a variety of difficulties with attention such as difficulties with response inhibition [21,22]. CPTs (Continues Performance Test) are widely used measures of attention. CPTs produce visual and auditory stimulating displays and measure the response to them, and have been used to support the clinician in asserting a diagnosis of ADHD in children with learning problems in the general population. Boys with Fragile X have difficulties in completing CPTs, even when compared with boys matched on their mental age. 40% of boys refused or were unable to complete a visual based CPT and 46% could not or would not complete an auditory CPT in a study by Sullivan et al. Mental age significantly predicted the ability of boys with Fragile X to complete a CPT. Failure of children with Fragile X (FXS) to complete the CPT was despite the writers efforts to simplify the task and design it for children with mental retardation [23]. In the 50-55% of boys with Fragile X who did complete the task, Sullivan documented initial difficulty in paying attention on both visual and auditory tasks but the boys were able to maintain attention consistently. Boys of the same mental age who did not have FXS showed deterioration of attention to task over time. This suggests that boys with Fragile X have more difficulty paying attention at the beginning of a task but are able to sustain their attention over time better than what would be expected from their developmental level. Performance of FXS boys was better on a visual based CPT. These findings have implications for educational planning. Of interest, in contrast with previous publications, inhibition skills for boys with Fragile X in this study were better than the sustained attention. Of note, 72% of the boys were taking psychotropic medication at the time of the assessment.

TREATMENT OF ADHD SYMPTOMS IN FRAGILE X

Children with Fragile X syndrome are commonly treated with a variety of medications for behavioral issues. In a caregiver report based study [20] 61% of males and 38% of females with Fragile X were taking medication; the most common symptoms treated were anxiety, attention and hyperactivity. Treatment for ADHD was common in childhood and declined substantially after the age of 18. Treatment for attention problems was reported for 37% of males and 23% of females and males. Individuals with FXS who were diagnosed with Autism were more likely to be treated for their hyperactivity. Parents perceived the medication their child was taking for attention hyperactivity was highly efficacious in about 25% of children and somewhat efficacious in an additional 40%. Despite the frequent use of medications aimed at ADHD symptoms with children with Fragile X, we found only one RCT that formally evaluated the effectiveness of common medications for ADHD. The study evaluated the effectiveness of Methylphenidate and amphetamines compared to placebo in a limited number of children. Methylphenidate was found to improve socialization skills and attention span in this small group [24]. Stimulants were found to have a significant response on inhibitory systems as measured by electrodermal response measures [16]

Because of growing literature that defines the molecular basis of FXS and better understanding cellular processes involved in the neurocognitive phenotype a number of medications thought to specifically enhance or inhibit intracellular processes have been studied as treatment of ADHD in boys with FXS in recent years. We will shortly introduce these studies in the following paragraphs.

L- acetylcarnitine (LAC) was examined in a double blind parallel multicenter study [25]. LAC is an acylated form of carnitine, an abundant ester in cerebral tissue and a target of research in a variety of neurological diseases, including ADHD [26]. In vitro, LAC has been shown to affect the FXS associated fragile site [27] and this was the rational for a clinical study. 63 patients were recruited to a double blind, placebo controlled, multi-center study. LAC treated patients showed greater reductions in the Connor's Global Index (both parents and teacher scales), although the difference did not reach statistical significance. LAC treated patients did improve in their overall behavior as measured on the Vineland Adaptive Scales. LAC in this study was well tolerated and drop out rate for the study was low (4 placebo and 3 LAC treated).

Minocycyline was examined as treatment for boys with Fragile X syndrome (FXS) in a few studies in recent years. Minocycline is a matrix metallo-protinase-9 (MMP-9) activity inhibitor. FMR1 knock-out mice treated with minocycline showed dendritic spine maturation and better behavioral performance then non treated mice [28]. MMP-9 activity is inhibited by FMRP. Minocycline reduces the high levels of MMP-9 activity in brains of mice models and FXS [28] and patients [29]. Paribello et al. [30] published the results of an open label treatment trial of Minocycline. Outcome measures were the Aberrant Behavior Checklist

/Community (ABC/C). The ABC is a 5 dimensional questionnaire that includes irritability, lethargy withdrawal, inappropriate speech, hyperactivity and stereotypic behavior. Statistically different improvements on the measures of irritability and stereotypy and hyperactive behavior were seen. In a randomized double blind placebo controlled trial of minocycline in children and adolescence with FXS the results were moderated and only the CGI- Clinical Global Impression scale improved after treatment as compared with placebo [31]. The study period was short (3 months) and due to the nature of the presumed activity of minocycline on neurons the researchers concluded that longer trials are indicated to further assess the benefits of minocycline in Fragile X. Studies in FMR1 knock-out mice also suggest that effect of minocycline will be longer-lasting in younger individuals [32].

Riluzole is hypothesized to have inhibitory effects on glutamate release, improving ERK activation as a measure of FMRP related glutamate disregulation. In a novel study by Erikson et al. [33] Riluzole was associated with improved ERK activation time, but clinically had a favorable effect on only 1 of 6 subjects. The relatively older age of the patient (young adults) the small number and the limited treatment duration were major study limitations, partly imposed by the high cost of Riluzole.

Valproic acid is a well-known antiepileptic drug also used as a mood stabilizer and in migraine therapy. It is an inhibitor of histone deacetylase (HDAC). Based on an in-vitro study that showed a modest reactivation of FMR1 transcription in lymphoblastoid cells treated with VPA, evaluation of VPA on ADHD symptoms in FXS patients was examined [34]. In the study be Toriolli et al. [35], 10 patients were enrolled in this study with a mean age of 10.6 years. Patients were treated for 6 months with a dose of up to 30 mg/kg/day. A trend towards a decrease in ADHD symptoms as measured on the Connors Parent Scales (Revised) was noted but the only statistically significant decrease was in the hyperactive symptom subscale. Study was mainly limited due to the small number of children and to its open label nature.

Glutamate receptor 5 modulators are currently being studied in a few multi-center large scale studies [36,37]

ADHD IN 22Q11.2 DELETION SYNDROME

22q11.2 deletion syndrome is the current accepted name of a group of genetic syndromes that previously were given names based on phenotypic findings that were varied. 22q11.2 deletion is the genetic deletion common to Velo-cardio-facial (Shprintzen) syndrome, Sedlackova syndrome, DiGeorge sequence, Cat eye syndrome or the acronym CATCH 22. Velo-cardio-facial syndrome received its name based on the findings unique facial futures and palatal abnormalities (particularly Velo-pharyngeal incompetence, submucosal cleft palate, and cleft palate-Shprinzen et al. 1978 [38]. The DiGeorge sequence (described by DiGeorge in the 1960s) described children that had the constellation of cardiovascular anomalies, hypoparathyroidism and absent thymus. Cat eye syndrome described children with facial abnormalities such as Preauricular tags and coloboma of the iris in addition to congenital heart defects. CATCH 22 was the acronym for children with Cardiac defects, Abnormal facies, Thymic hypoplasia, Cleft palate and Hypocalcemia.

Most cases of 22q11.2 deletion syndrome have a 3 mega based deletion encompassing a region containing 40 genes. Less than 10% of cases have a smaller deletion. It is estimated that the incidence 22q11.2 deletion syndrome ranges from 1 per 2000 to 1 per 4000 people in the general population [39]. An estimated 90% of individuals with 22q11 deletion have a De-novo deletion but approximately 10% carry a familial abnormality which is transferred as an autosomal dominant trait. 22q11.2 deletion is the second most common genetic finding in children with a congenital heart defect, ranging from 5% [40] to 15% [41]. 22q11.2 deletion is detected in 20% of children with conotruncal heart defects in general, and in 50% of those with an interrupted aortic arch [42,43].

Despite the common findings of major anomalies n children with 22q11.2 deletion, not all children have such a diagnosis. In fact congenital heart defects are present in only 74% of individuals genetically diagnosed with 22q11.2 deletion. The most common heart anomaly in 22q11.2 deficiency is a Ventricular Septal Defect (VSD). Palatial abnormalities are found in 69% [44] of individuals diagnosed with 22q11.2 deletion. The most common form of palatal anomaly is not the classical cleft palate as described in the past [38] but rather a submucosal cleft palate or occult submucosal cleft palate. These clefts are difficult to identify without specific procedures such as a nasopharyngoscopy. Velopharngeal insufficiency may be the only palatial finding (So called Sedlackova syndrome), and hypernasal speech has been described in some cases with 22q11.2 deletion that were undiagnosed for a long time [45]. An immune deficiency is common and affects about 77% of individuals with 22q11 deficiency although the clinical presentation is varied and may be very mild. The "complete" DiGeorge syndrome with total absence of the thymus and the severe T cell immune deficiency accounts for less 0.5 of the patients. The majority of patients with 22q11 deletion have a partial defect with impaired thymic development, variable defects in T cell numbers and, in some individuals, humeral deficiencies [46]. Hypocalcaemia is another common presentation in childhood (50%).

Developmental delays are in fact the most common characteristic associated with 22q11.2 deletion and effect 70% to 90% of individuals [44]. The majority of children with 22q11 deletion have lower than normal IQs. As a group, IQ in is in the low borderline range, with a bell shaped distribution around the mean. Mild mental retardation is very common and severe MR is rare. In one of the largest studies published in recent years by Niklasson et al. 2009 [47], a hundred individuals with 22q11 deficiencies participated with a mean IQ of 71, 42% mild MR in IQ range of 50 to 70. Females had a slightly higher mean IQ than males (IQ75/IQ65).

Psychiatric disorders have frequently been described in individuals with 22q11.2 deletions. Schizophrenia may be dramatic presenting feature of individuals with 22q11.2 deletion [48]. Schizophrenia has been reported to occur in 1% (in children and adolescents, [49]) to 11% [50], but psychotic symptoms are more common and have been observed in 14-28% of children [49].

Anxiety is the most common psychiatric disorder in subjects with 22q11/2del and was reported in 39% of 323 individuals pooled from 7 studies in a review by Jolin et al. 2012 [51].

ADHD is the second most frequent psychiatric disorder in children with 22q11.2 deletion with a rate of 38% [51]. The occurrence of ADHD varied from 12% to 46% across the 7 studies reviewed. In a study that included children only (N=30, age 7 to 13 years), ADHD was diagnosed in 13 children. The presence the diagnosis of ADHD was based on an interview, using the DSM4, the Conners Brief Parent Questionnaire and the CBCL. Full scale IQ was 72.1 (range 46 to 94). In this group there was a high prevalence of autism spectrum disorder (8 of 30) and half of the children with a diagnosis of ASD had a concurrent diagnosis of ADHD. In children with ADHD and ASD, IQ was significantly lower with a mean of 59.3. Inattention was a prominent feature in children with 22q11 deficiency. The diagnosis of ADHD did consider the low intellectual level of the children.

Autism Spectrum Disorder is another common neuropsychiatric disorder in 22q11.1 deletion syndrome, described in 20% [52] to 50% [53] of children.

Because childhood anxiety, schizophrenia, autism spectrum disorder and ADHD share many features, and because some children may have comorbidities, the diagnosis of ADHD in these children may be even more difficult then in other disorders of ID described previously. Therefore a thorough developmental and psychiatric evaluation should be carried out for young children and adolescents with 22q11.2 deletion syndrome and behavioral difficulties, and they should be followed by a multidisciplinary team as new issues may arise during adolescence.

TREATMENT OF ADHD IN CHILDREN WITH 22Q11.2 DELETION

Data specifically regarding the use of medications to treat ADHD symptoms in children with 22q11 deletion is limited. Gothelf et al. (2003) [54] reported significant improvement of symptoms in an open label trial of MPH, and similar results in randomized controlled trial [55]. In the RCT study, the primary outcome was an executive function task ("Heart and flowers") and a CPT after a single administration of MPH. A more clinically relevant 6 month follow up visit showed a significant reduction in severity of ADHD symptoms as reported on the Connors parent rating scale.

Catechol-O-Methionine tranferase (COMT) is a gene that resides in the deletion area in 22q11.2del syndrome. COMT encodes for an enzymes that is involved in dopamine degradation. Reduced COMT activity has been suggested in the pathophysiology of the neuropsychiatric abnormalities in individuals with 22q11.2 syndrome [56]. A pioneering study of S-Adenosyl-L-Methionine (SAMe), which enhances activity of COMT enzyme, was conducted. The study was a 6 week RCT that assessed both depressive and ADHD symptoms. No significant benefits were detected [57]

Interestingly, CXCR4 which is a key regulator of interneuron migration, was recently shown to be reduced in a mouse models of 22q11.2 deletion [58,59]. This finding may be a key to targeted medications as currently there are specific antibodies for CXCR4 that have been shown to have clinical effect in other medical conditions [60,61]

ADHD IN NEUROFIBROMATOSIS 1
(VON RECKLINGHAUSEN DISEASE)

Neurofibromatosis type 1 (NF1) is one of the most common neurocutaneous disorders, with a prevalence of about 1 in 3,000. It is an autosomal dominant hereditary condition, although approximately half of all cases are caused by spontaneous mutations. Mutations within NF1 gene (17q11.2) result in loss of function of the protein neurofibromin leading to increase cell proliferation and tumorgenesis. NF1 is clinically diagnosed when 2 of 7 criteria are met (Café-au-lait spots, neurofibromas, freckling, optic tract gliomas, Lisch nodules, distinctive osseous lesions, family history). Sequencing of the neurofibromin gene is the preferred molecular diagnostic study, detecting >95% of affected individuals. Neoplasms and vascular disease contribute to the shorter life expectancy (mean 54 years) of individuals affected by NF1 [62], but most patients will live well into adulthood.

Intellectual disability is not sine-qua-non with NF1. IQ< 70 has been reported to affect less then 10% of individuals affected by NF1 [63,64]. The average IQ is shifted downward, and a 1/3 of patients have an IQ that is less then average [65]. Differences in intellectual functioning can be detected in early preschool years. In a cohort of 3 year old children with NF1, the average full scale IQ was 96.2 (Controls in this study had a FSIQ of 112, [66]). The average IQ in a cohort of older patients was 88.6 (101.6 in the control group) [63]. Neurological and medical complications are weakly associated with lower full scale IQ. Gross deletions of the NF1 gene are associated with a more severe phenotype, including dysmorphic features, developmental delay and learning disability [67]. The molecular mechanism that underlies the cognitive and behavioural deficits in NF1 is thought to be related to increased Ras function due to loss of inhibition by neurofibromin [68].

Although not all individuals with NF1 have a developmental disability by definition, academic impairment is a frequent finding in children and adolescents with NF1 and can affect more then 60% of them [69]. In the following paragraphs we will try to delineate the type of academic impairments and the effect of ADHD symptomology on school performance in children with NF1.

Early work on school difficulties in children with NF1 recognized the unique neuropsychological profile. In a 1997 consensus statement [70], children with NF1 were regarded as having learning disabilities, and these were stated as "a major discrepancy between ability (intellect or aptitude) and achievement (performance)". The guidelines for management of learning issues in children included early discussion with parents as part of the medical assessment. Developmental history and review of school progress were recommended, and "attentional deficits" acknowledged. This was based a literature that consistently measures "attention problems" affecting up to 50% of children [71].

Hyman et al. (2006) [72] found that although 52% of children with NF1 in their cohort had problems with academic achievement, only 20% of the children could formally receive a diagnosis of a specific learning disability (SLD). The study group defined three subtypes of learning profiles in children with NF1: One with a formal SLD (20%), a group with general lowered IQ (GLD- General Learning Difficulties, 30% of group), and those without learning difficulties (48%). The researchers specifically addressed the question of inattention in the cohort. All three groups had a high rate of ADHD. The group with a literacy based SLD had the highest rate of ADHD (70%). Children with GLD had an ADHD rate of 46%. All groups performed below norm on visuospatial tests.

Pride et al. (2012) [73] compared cognitive functioning and academic achievement between a group of children with NF1 with or without ADHD. Their results showed that the inattention and executive dysfunction significantly undermined academic achievement in children with NF1. Although both groups, on average, had a full scale IQ that was lower than normative mean, IQ in children with NF1 without ADHD was significantly higher than children with NF1 and ADHD. This finding was corroborated by another recent study by Lidzba et al. [65].

Following the establishment of the relationship between NF1, cognition, SLD and ADHD, specific aspects of attention were investigated. In a cohort of 55 school aged children,

42% were diagnosed with ADHD, consistent with previous work [74]. ADHD subtypes were found to be as follows: 20% predominantly inattentive type, 40% predominantly hyperactive/ impulsive type and 40% with a combined type. These findings differ from "non syndromic" ADHD, where predominantly inattentive ADHD is the most common subtype [75]. In Isenberg's study, children with NF1, with or without ADHD, performed significantly lower on a variety of tests such as tests of sustained auditory attention, divided auditory attention and a CPT. The authors concluded that measures for normative populations, such as the DSM4, do not fully capture all the attention problems experienced by children with NF1, resulting in a failure to identify children with NF1 who would benefit from appropriate interventions. Payne et al. (2012) [76] compared children's function on measures of spatial working memory and inhibition control and found that in children with NF1, with or without ADHD, executive function as impaired. The researcher's interpretation of the results was that executive dysfunction is not a unique contributor to ADHD symptomology in children with NF1.

ADHD can persist through adulthood and effects quality of life. This was found true for adults with NF1 as well, and those with NF1 and ADHD reported having lower life satisfaction with symptoms affecting self-satisfaction, sexuality and family [77] then adults with NF1/no ADHD.

TREATMENT OF ADHD IN NF1

In 2002 Mautner et al. reported that low doses (5-15 mg) of methylphenidate improved TOVA scores in a group of school aged children with NF1 [71], and significantly improved CBCL sores in a 1 year follow up. The main flaw of this study was that it was not an RCT. Reliability of TOVA as a single measure of ADHD symptoms has also been questioned in recent years. No other studies examining the efficacy of MPH in NF1 have been published, and therefore the findings have not been replicated in any other study.

New findings supporting Mautner's report came from a recent study in a novel NF1 mouse model. In the study, NF1 optic glioma genetically engineered mice (OPG-GEM) exhibited defects in attention without accompanying hyperactivity as measured by abnormal locomotor activity levels and abnormal exploratory behaviors. These mice had reduced dopamine levels in the striatum, and administration of methylphenidate reversed their clinical ADHD phenotype [78].

The finding of favorable response to MPH have been challenged in the study described above by Isenberg et al. Isenberg's study group was divided into 2 subgroups based on whether they were receiving or not receiving stimulant medication, and the results were that the group of children who were diagnosed with ADHD and were on medications (approximately 25% of children with NF1 and ADHD) received the same scores on the Connors parent ratings as those who were not medicated at the time. There were no significant differences between the medicated/non medicated groups within scores on various subscales of the Connors third edition parents rating. Notably parent responding to the Connors questionnaire indicated that children on stimulant medication were more inattentive and oppositional then children not on medications.

In 2002, Costa et al. reported that in mice models of NF1, GABA-mediated inhibition is increased and causes deficits in long term potentiation. Increased GABA inhibition is controlled in NF1 by excessive Ras activity, which normally is suppressed by neurofibromin. Lovastatin, a potential inhibitor of p21Ras, was shown rescue long term potentiation deficit and to reverse spatial learning and attention deficits in a mouse model [79]. Treatment with Lovastatin had an affect on resting state functional connectivity (RSFG) as measured by 3-T echo-planar-imaging (fMRI technique) in 7 children with NF1 [80]. Despite these promising trials, two RCTs with simvastatin did not show any affect on cognitive deficits or behavioral problems [81,82]

RISPERIDONE FOR CHILDREN WITH ID AND ADHD DISRUPTIVE BEHAVIOUR

Risperidone is an atypical antipsychotic drug that is FDA approved for the treatment of schizophrenia, bipolar disorder and irritability in autistic disorder. Risperidone has been used in children with ID to reduce aggression and hyperactivity in both open label and placebo controlled trials in recent years [83,84]. The addition of risperidone to a psychostimulant resulted in significantly better control of hyperactivity than was achieved with stimulant treatment alone in a follow-up study of the original ID group [85]. In a head-to-head trial of methylphenidate vs. risperidone for treatment of ADHD, risperidone was associated with greater reductions in ADHD than methylphenidate in children with moderate mental retardation and ADHD [86].

Risperidone has some serious side effects. It is most commonly associated with metabolic changes that may increase cardiovascular/cerebrovascular risk. These metabolic changes include hyperglycemia, dyslipidemia, and significant weight gain. Less common but potential side effects are neuroleptic malignant syndrome and tardive dyskinesia. Due to this, it is usually prudent to try stimulants before antipsychotics in children with ID and ADHD with severe disruptive behavior.

CONCLUSION

Symptoms of ADHD have been frequently observed in children with ID and traditionally have been considered by clinicians and researchers to be consistent with the delayed developmental age. In recent years, there is increasing evidence to support the validity of making a diagnosis of ADHD in people with ID. Moreover, children with genetic syndromes that cause ID appear to have unique ADHD profiles e.g., the hyperactivity and aggression that are common in FXS vs. the severe impairment in executive function in children with NF1. The relationship between IQ and ADHD is complex, and while in some syndromes ADHD is not correlated to IQ (e.g., Down syndrome), in others it is not clear whether the ADHD affects cognition or both impairments are a result of the same neuropathological process in a more severe presentation.

Identification of ADHD may frequently be difficult due to the need to differentiate ADHD from other neurocognitive diagnoses that occur in these syndromes such as ID vs. a specific learning disability or autism spectrum disorder. In addition, there is a high rate of comorbidity of these conditions in the common genetic syndromes described.

Symptoms of ADHD may be the presenting symptoms of a genetic syndrome prior to the identification of developmental delay, especially in the syndromes where the hyperactive/impulsive type is common such as fragile X. It is therefore advised that children with ADHD and developmental delay, dysmorphic features or neurocutaneus markings be referred to a pediatric developmental center for a full evaluation of their behavioral and cognitive abilities and related medical issues that may mimic or exacerbate ADHD (e.g., low visual acuity in Down syndrome).

Identifying symptoms of ADHD, making an appropriate differential diagnosis and diagnosing ADHD and comorbidities in children with ID is vital, because ADHD may result in decreased ability to participate in learning situations. For instance, a child with Down syndrome and behavioral problems may be frequently removed from a learning situation even if the learning pace is appropriate for his level of cognitive impairment. A child with fragile X may not be having hyperactive symptoms but may have difficulty initiating attention on a task, missing many learning opportunities within a small and supportive classroom. We have shown that identification of the type of ADHD and even more specifically areas of strengths and weaknesses within ADHD domains can support school planning (e.g., using more visual then auditory materials to present new material to a child).

Little is known on the effect of common medications such as methylphenidate or amphetamines for treatment of ADHD in children with ID. Few high level studies have been attempted, and no clinical trials with atomoxetine were published in pubmed to date. Those studies that have been done showed good response to MPH, but data coming out of non-clinical trials is at times equivocal. Because mechanisms of abnormal brain development in children with ID are unique for each syndrome, it is unlikely that the pathways in which amphetamines influence ADHD in cognitively intact children and children with ID are identical, and therefore differences in response are expected.

As the molecular and cellular aspects of a variety of syndrome unveils before us, we hope to learn more about potential specific medications that will support cognitive development and decrease related unwanted behaviors in genetic syndromes that cause ID.

REFERENCES

[1]   Maulik PK, Mascarenhas MN, Mathers CD, Dua T, Saxena S. Prevalence of intellectual disability: a meta-analysis of population-based studies. *Res Dev Disabil.* 2011;32:419-36.

[2]   Coleen A. Boyle, Sheree Boulet, Laura A. Schieve, Robin A. Cohen, Stephen J. Trends in the Prevalence of Developmental Disabilities in US Children, 1997-2008. *Pediatrics.* 2011;127:1034-42 .

[3]   Ekstein S, Glick B, Weill M, Kay B, Berger I. Down syndrome and attention-deficit/hyperactivity disorder (ADHD). *J Child Neurol.* 2011;26:1290-5.

[4]   Thomson A, Maltezos S, Paliokosta E, Xenitidis K. Amfetamine for attention deficit hyperactivity disorder in people with intellectual disabilities. *Cochrane Database Syst Rev.* 2009 ;21

[5]   Fox RA, Wade EJ. Attention deficit hyperactivity disorder among adults with severe and profound mental retardation. *Res Dev Disabil.* 1998;19:275-80.

[6]   Antshel KM, Phillips MH, Gordon M, Barkley R, Faraone SV. Is ADHD a valid disorder in children with intellectual delays? *Clin Psychol Rev.* 2006;26:555-72.

[7]   Hastings RP, Beck A, Daley D, Hill C. Symptoms of ADHD and their correlates in children with intellectual disabilities.*Res Dev Disabil.* 2005;26:456-68.

[8]   Sullivan K, Hatton D, Hammer J, Sideris J, Hooper S, Ornstein P, Bailey D Jr. ADHD symptoms in children with FXS. *Am J Med Genet A.* 2006;140:2275-88.

[9]   Cornish K, Steele A, Monteiro CR, Karmiloff-Smith A, Scerif G.Blumberg, Marshalyn Yeargin-Allsopp, Susanna Visser and Michael D. Kogan. Attention deficits predict phenotypic outcomes in syndrome-specific and domain-specific ways. *Front Psychol.* 2012;11:3:227.

[10]   Baird PA, Sadovnick AD. Life tables for Down syndrome. *Hum Genet.*1989;82:291-2.

[11]   Weijerman ME, de Winter JP. Clinical practice. The care of children with Down syndrome. *Eur J Pediatr.* 2010;169:1445-52. doi: 10.1007/s00431-010-1253-0. Epub 2010 Jul 15.

[12]   Prevalence of Down Syndrome Among Children and Adolescents in 10 Regions of the United States. *Pediatrics* 2009;1565-1571.

[13]   Capone G, Goyal P, Ares W, Lannigan E. Neurobehavioral disorders in children, adolescents, and young adults with Down syndrome. *Am J Med Genet C Semin Med Genet.* 2006; 142C:158-72.

[14]   Coe DA, Matson JL, Russell DW, Slifer KJ, Capone GT, Baglio C, Stallings S. Behavior problems of children with Down syndrome and life events. *J Autism Dev Disord.* 1999;29:149-56.

[15]   Schneider A, Hagerman RJ, Hessl D. Fragile X syndrome -- from genes to cognition. *Dev Disabil Res Rev.* 2009;15:333-42.

[16]   Hagerman RJ, Miller LJ, McGrath-Clarke J, Riley K, Goldson E, Harris SW, Simon J, Church K, Bonnell J, Ognibene TC, McIntosh DN. Influence of stimulants on electrodermal studies in Fragile X syndrome. *Microsc Res Tech.* 2002;57:168-73.

[17]   Moon J, Beaudin AE, Verosky S, Driscoll LL, Weiskopf M, Levitsky DA, Crnic LS,Strupp BJ. Attentional dysfunction, impulsivity, and resistance to change in a mouse model of fragile X syndrome. *Behav Neurosci.* 2006;120:1367-79.

[18]   Hagerman R, Kemper M, Hudson M. Learning disabilities and attentional problems in boys with the fragile X syndrome. *Am J Dis Child.* 1985;139:674-8.

[19]   Farzin F, Perry H, Hessl D, Loesch D, Cohen J, Bacalman S, Gane L, Tassone F, Hagerman P, Hagerman R. Autism spectrum disorders and attention-deficit/hyperactivity disorder in boys with the fragile X premutation. *J Dev Behav Pediatr.* 2006;27:S137-44.

[20]   Bailey DB Jr, Raspa M, Bishop E, Olmsted M, Mallya UG, Berry-Kravis E. Medication utilization for targeted symptoms in children and adults with fragile X syndrome: US survey. *J Dev Behav Pediatr.* 2012;33:62-9.

[21]   Munir F, Cornish KM, Wilding J. Nature of the working memory deficit in fragile-X syndrome. *Brain Cogn.* 2000;44:387-401.

[22]   Wilding J, Cornish K, Munir F. Further delineation of the executive deficit in males with fragile-X syndrome. *Neuropsychologia.* 2002;40:1343-9.

[23] Sullivan K, Hatton DD, Hammer J, Sideris J, Hooper S, Ornstein PA, Bailey DB Jr. Sustained attention and response inhibition in boys with fragile X syndrome: measures of continuous performance. *Am J Med Genet B Neuropsychiatr Genet.* 2007.

[24] Hagerman RJ, Murphy MA, Wittenberger MD. A controlled trial of stimulant medication in children with the fragile X syndrome. *Am J Med Genet.*1988;30:377-92.

[25] Torrioli MG, Vernacotola S, Peruzzi L, Tabolacci E, Mila M, Militerni R, Musumeci S, Ramos FJ, Frontera M, Sorge G, Marzullo E, Romeo G, Vallee L, Veneselli E, Cocchi E, Garbarino E, Moscato U, Chiurazzi P, D'Iddio S, Calvani M, Neri G. A double-blind, parallel, multicenter comparison of L-acetylcarnitine with placebo on the attention deficit hyperactivity disorder in fragile X syndrome boys. *Am J Med Genet A.* 2008;146:803-12. doi:10.1002/ajmg.a.32268. PubMed PMID: 18286595.

[26] Van Oudheusden LJ, Scholte Efficacy of carnitine in the treatment of children with attention-deficit hyperactivity disorder. *HR Prostaglandins Leukot Essent Fatty Acids.* 2002;67:33-8.

[27] Pomponi MG, Neri G. Butyrate and acetyl-carnitine inhibit the cytogenetic expression of the fragile X in vitro. *Am J Med Genet.* 1994;15;51:447-50.

[28] Bilousova TV, Dansie L, Ngo M, Aye J, Charles JR, Ethell DW, Ethell IM. Minocycline promotes dendritic spine maturation and improves behavioural performance in the fragile X mouse model. *J Med Genet.* 2009;46:94-102. doi: 10.1136/jmg.2008.061796

[29] Dziembowska M, Pretto DI, Janusz A, Kaczmarek L, Leigh MJ, Gabriel N, Durbin-Johnson B, Hagerman RJ, Tassone F. High MMP-9 activity levels in fragile X syndrome are lowered by minocycline. *Am J Med Genet A.* 2013;161A:1897-903. doi: 10.1002/ajmg.a.36023

[30] Paribello C, Tao L, Folino A, Berry-Kravis E, Tranfaglia M, Ethell IM, Ethell DW. Open label add-on treatment trial of minocycline in fragile X syndrome. *BMC Neurol.* 2010;10:91. doi: 10.1186/1471-2377-10-91. PubMed PMID: 2093712.

[31] Leigh MJ, Nguyen DV, Mu Y, Winarni TI, Schneider A, Chechi T, Polussa J, Doucet P, Tassone F, Rivera SM, Hessl D, Hagerman RJ. A randomized double-blind, placebo-controlled trial of minocycline in children and adolescents with fragile x syndrome. *J Dev Behav Pediatr.* 2013;34:147-55. doi: 10.1097/DBP.0b013e318287cd17

[32] Dansie LE, Phommahaxay K, Okusanya AG, Uwadia J, Huang M, Rotschafer SE, Razak KA, Ethell DW, Ethell IM. Long-lasting effects of minocycline on behavior in young but not adult Fragile X mice. *Neuroscience.* 2013;246:186-98. doi: 10.1016/j.neuroscience.2013.04.058. Epub 2013 May 7.

[33] Erickson CA, Weng N, Weiler IJ, Greenough WT, Stigler KA, Wink LK, McDougle CJ. Open-label riluzole in fragile X syndrome. *Brain Res.* 2011; 70-1380:264;22doi: 10.1016/j.brainres.2010.10.108. Epub 2010 Nov 5. PubMed PMID: 21059347.

[34] Tabolacci E, De Pascalis I, Accadia M, Terracciano A, Moscato U, Chiurazzi P, Neri G.Modest reactivation of the mutant FMR1 gene by valproic acid is accompanied by histone modifications but not DNA demethylation. *Pharmacogenet Genomics.* 2008;18:738-41. doi: 10.1097/FPC.0b013e32830500a1.

[35] Torrioli M, Vernacotola S, Setini C, Bevilacqua F, Martinelli D, Snape M, Hutchison JA, Di Raimo FR, Tabolacci E, Neri G. Treatment with valproic acid ameliorates ADHD symptoms in fragile X syndrome boys. *Am J Med Genet A.* 2010;152A:1420-7. doi: 10.1002/ajmg.a.33484. PubMed PMID: 20503316.

[36] Osterweil EK, Krueger DD, Reinhold K, Bear MF .Hypersensitivity to mGluR5 and ERK1/2 leads to excessive protein synthesis in the hippocampus of a mouse model of fragile X syndrome. *J Neurosci.* 2010 ;30:15616-27. doi: 10.1523/JNEUROSCI.3888-10.20.

[37] Burket JA, Herndon AL, Winebarger EE, Jacome LF, Deutsch SI. 10. Complex effects of mGluR5 antagonism on sociability and stereotypic behaviors in mice: possible implications for the pharmacotherapy of autism spectrum disorders. *Brain Res Bull.* 2011 ;86:152-8. doi: 10.1016.

[38] Shprintzen RJ, Goldberg RB, Lewin ML, Sidoti EJ, Berkman MD, Argamaso RV, Young D. A new syndrome involving cleft palate, cardiac anomalies, typical facies, and learning disabilities: velo-cardio-facial syndrome. *Cleft Palate J.* 1978;15:56-62.

[39] Shprintzen RJ. Velo-cardio-facial syndrome: 30 Years of study. *Dev Disabil Res Rev.* 2008;14:3-10. doi: 10.1002/ddrr.2

[40] Tomita-Mitchell A, Mahnke DK, Larson JM, Ghanta S, Feng Y, Simpson PM, Broeckel U, Duffy K, Tweddell JS, Grossman WJ, Routes JM, Mitchell ME. Multiplexed quantitative real-time PCR to detect 22q11.2 deletion in patients with congenital heart disease. *Physiol Genomics.* 2010;42A:52-60. doi: 10.1152/physiolgenomics.00073.2010.

[41] Wozniak A, Wolnik-Brzozowska D, Wisniewska M, Glazar R, Materna-Kiryluk A, Moszura T, Badura-Stronka M, Skolozdrzy J, Krawczynski MR, Zeyland J, Bobkowski W, Slomski R, Latos-Bielenska A, Siwinska A. Frequency of 22q11.2 microdeletion in children with congenital heart defects in western poland. *BMC Pediatr.* 2010;10:88. doi: 10.1186/1471-2431-10-88.

[42] Halder A, Jain M, Chaudhary I, Kabra M. Prevalence of 22q11.2 microdeletion in 146 patients with cardiac malformation in a referral hospital of North India. *BMC Med Genet.* 2010 ;11:101. doi: 10.1186/1471-2350-11-101.

[43] Goldmuntz E, Clark BJ, Mitchell LE, Jawad AF, Cuneo BF, Reed L, McDonald-McGinn D, Chien P, Feuer J, Zackai EH, Emanuel BS, Driscoll DA.Frequency of 22q11 deletions in patients with conotruncal defects. *J Am Coll Cardiol.* 1998;32:492-8.

[44] McDonald-McGinn DM, Sullivan KE. *Chromosome 22q11.2 deletion syndrome (DiGeorge syndrome/velocardiofacial syndrome Medicine (Baltimore).* 2011;90:1-18. doi: 10.1097/MD.0b013e3182060469. Review.

[45] Beaujard MP, Chantot S, Dubois M, Keren B, Carpentier W, Mabboux P, Whalen S, Vodovar M, Siffroi JP, Portnoï MF. Atypical deletion of 22q11.2: detection using the FISH TBX1 probe and molecular characterization with high-density SNP arrays. *Eur J Med Genet.* 2009;52:321-7. doi: 10.1016/j.ejmg.2009.05.010. Epub 2009 May 23.

[46] McLean-Tooke A, Barge D, Spickett GP, Gennery AR. *J Allergy Clin Immunol.* 2008;122:362-7, 367.e1-4. doi: 10.1016/j.jaci.2008.03.033. Immunologic defects in 22q11.2 deletion syndrome.

[47] Niklasson L, Gillberg C. The neuropsychology of 22q11 deletion syndrome. A neuropsychiatric study of 100 individuals. *Res Dev Disabil.* 2010;31:185-94. doi: 10.1016/j.ridd.2009.09.001

[48] Kook SD, An SK, Kim KR, Kim WJ, Lee E, Namkoong K.. Psychotic features as the first manifestation of 22q11.2 deletion syndrome. *Psychiatry Investig.* 2010;7:72-4. doi: 10.4306/pi.2010.7.1.72. Epub 2010 Feb 19.

[49] Jolin EM, Weller RA, Jessani NR, Zackai EH, McDonald-McGinn DM, Weller EB.Affective disorders and other psychiatric diagnoses in children and adolescents with 22q11.2 Deletion Syndrome. *J Affect Disord.* 2009;119:177-80. doi: 10.1016/j.jad.2009.02.016

[50] Tang SX, Yi JJ, Calkins ME, Whinna DA, Kohler CG, Souders MC, McDonald-McGinn DM, Zackai EH, Emanuel BS, Gur RC, Gur RE. Psychiatric disorders in 22q11.2 deletion syndrome are prevalent but undertreated. *Psychol Med.* 2013;9:1-11.

[51] Jolin EM, Weller RA, Weller EB.Occurrence of affective disorders compared to other psychiatric disorders in children and adolescents with 22q11.2 deletion syndrome. *J Affect Disord.* 2012;136:222-8. doi: 10.1016/j.jad.2010.11.025.

[52] Antshel KM, Aneja A, Strunge L, Peebles J, Fremont WP, Stallone K, Abdulsabur N, Higgins AM, Shprintzen RJ, Kates WR. Autistic spectrum disorders in velo-cardio facial syndrome (22q11.2 deletion). *J Autism Dev Disord.* 2007;37:1776-86.

[53] Vorstman JA, Morcus ME, Duijff SN, Klaassen PW, Heineman-de Boer JA, Beemer FA, Swaab H, Kahn RS, van Engeland H. The 22q11.2 deletion in children: high rate of autistic disorders and early onset of psychotic symptoms. *J Am Acad Child Adolesc Psychiatry.* 2006;45:1104-13.

[54] Gothelf D, Gruber R, Presburger G, Dotan I, Brand-Gothelf A, Burg M, Inbar D, Steinberg T, Frisch A, Apter A, Weizman A. Methylphenidate treatment for attention-deficit/hyperactivity disorder in children and adolescents with velocardiofacial syndrome: an open-label study. *J Clin Psychiatry.* 2003;64:1163-9. PubMed PMID: 14658963.C

[55] Green T, Weinberger R, Diamond A, Berant M, Hirschfeld L, Frisch A, Zarchi O,Weizman A, Gothelf D. The effect of methylphenidate on prefrontal cognitivefunctioning, inattention, and hyperactivity in velocardiofacial syndrome. *J Child Adolesc Psychopharmacol.* 2011;21:589-95. doi: 10.1089/cap.2011.0042. Epub 2011 Dec 7. PubMed PMID: 22149470.

[56] Armando M, Papaleo F, Vicari S. COMT implication in cognitive and psychiatric symptoms in chromosome 22q11 microdeletion syndrome: a selective review. *CNS Neurol Disord Drug Targets.* 2012;11:273-81

[57] Green T, Steingart L, Frisch A, Zarchi O, Weizman A, Gothelf D. The feasibility and safety of S-adenosyl-L-methionine (SAMe) for the treatment of neuropsychiatric symptoms in 22q11.2 deletion syndrome: a double-blind placebo-controlled trial. *J Neural Transm.* 2012;119:1417-23. doi: 10.1007/s00702-012-0831-x. Epub 2012 Jun 8.

[58] Toritsuka M, Kimoto S, Muraki K, Landek-Salgado MA, Yoshida A, Yamamoto N, Horiuchi Y, Hiyama H, Tajinda K, Keni N, Illingworth E, Iwamoto T, Kishimoto T, Sawa A, Tanigaki K. Deficits in microRNA-mediated Cxcr4/Cxcl12 signaling in neurodevelopmental deficits in a 22q11 deletion syndrome mouse model. *Proc Natl Acad Sci U S A.* 2013;110:17552-7. doi: 10.1073/pnas.1312661110. Epub 2013 Oct 7. PMID:24101523

[59] Meechan DW, Tucker ES, Maynard TM, LaMantia AS. Cxcr4 regulation of interneuron migration is disrupted in 22q11.2 deletion syndrome. *Proc Natl Acad Sci U S A.* 2012 ;109:18601-6. doi: 10.1073/pnas.1211507109. Epub 2012 Oct 22.

[60] McDermott DH, Liu Q, Ulrick J, Kwatemaa N, Anaya-O'Brien S, Penzak SR, Filho JO, Priel DA, Kelly C, Garofalo M, Littel P, Marquesen MM, Hilligoss D, Decastro R, Fleisher TA, Kuhns DB, Malech HL, Murphy PM. The CXCR4 antagonist plerixafor

corrects panleukopenia in patients with WHIM syndrome. *Blood.* 2011 ;118:4957-62. doi: 10.1182/blood-2011-07-368084. Epub 2011 Sep 2.

[61] Uy GL, Rettig MP, Motabi IH, McFarland K, Trinkaus KM, Hladnik LM, Kulkarni S, Abboud CN, Cashen AF, Stockerl-Goldstein KE, Vij R, Westervelt P, DiPersio JF. A phase 1/2 study of chemosensitization with the CXCR4 antagonist plerixafor in relapsed or refractory acute myeloid leukemia. *Blood.* 2012 ;119:3917-24. doi: 10.1182/blood-2011-10-383406

[62] Rasmussen SA, Yang Q, Friedman JM. Mortality in neurofibromatosis 1: an analysis using U.S. death certificates. Am J Hum Genet. 2001;68:1110-8. Epub 2001 Mar 28.

[63] Ferner RE, Hughes RA, Weinman J. Intellectual impairment in neurofibromatosis 1. *J Neurol Sci.* 1996;138:125-33.

[64] Hyman SL, Shores A, North KN. The nature and frequency of cognitive deficits in children with neurofibromatosis type 1. *Neurology.* 2005 ;65:1037-44.

[65] Lidzba K, Granström S, Lindenau J, Mautner VF. The adverse influence of attention-deficit disorder with or without hyperactivity on cognition in neurofibromatosis type 1. *Dev Med Child Neurol.* 2012;54:892-7. doi: 10.1111/j.1469-8749.2012.04377.x. Epub 2012 Aug 9. PubMed PMID: 22881119.

[66] .Lorenzo J, Barton B, Arnold SS, North KN. Cognitive features that distinguish preschool-age children with neurofibromatosis type 1 from their peers: a matched case-control study. *J Pediatr.* 2013;163:1479-83.e1. doi: 10.1016/j.jpeds.2013.06.038. Epub 2013 Aug 1.

[67] Upadhyaya M, Ruggieri M, Maynard J, Osborn M, Hartog C, Mudd S, Penttinen M, Cordeiro I, Ponder M, Ponder BA, Krawczak M, Cooper DN. Gross deletions of the neurofibromatosis type 1 (NF1) gene are predominantly of maternal origin and commonly associated with a learning disability, dysmorphic features and developmental delay .Hum Genet. 1998;102:591-7.

[68] Costa RM, Silva AJ. Molecular and cellular mechanisms underlying the cognitive deficits associated with neurofibromatosis 1. *J Child Neurol.* 2002;17:622-6.

[69] Coudé FX, Mignot C, Lyonnet S, Munnich A. Academic impairment is the most frequent complication of neurofibromatosis type-1 (NF1) in children. *Behav Genet.* 2006;36:660-4.

[70] North KN, Riccardi V, Samango-Sprouse C, Ferner R, Moore B, Legius E, Ratner N, Denckla MB. Cognitive function and academic performance in neurofibromatosis. 1: consensus statement from the NF1 Cognitive Disorders Task Force. *Neurology.* 1997;48:1121-7.

[71] Mautner VF, Kluwe L, Thakker SD, Leark RA. Treatment of ADHD in neurofibromatosis type 1. *Dev Med Child Neurol.* 2002;44:164-70.

[72] Hyman SL, Arthur Shores E, North KN. Learning disabilities in children with neurofibromatosis type 1: subtypes, cognitive profile, and attention-deficit-hyperactivity disorder. *Dev Med Child Neurol.* 2006;48:973-7. PubMed PMID: 17109785

[73] Pride NA, Payne JM, North KN. The impact of ADHD on the cognitive and academic functioning of children with NF1. *Dev Neuropsychol.* 2012;37:590-600 doi: 10.1080/87565641.2012.695831. PubMed PMID: 23066937.

[74]   Isenberg JC, Templer A, Gao F, Titus JB, Gutmann DH. Attention skills in children
       with   neurofibromatosis   type   1.   *J   Child   Neurol.*   2013;28:45-9.   doi:
       10.1177/0883073812439435. Epub 2012 Apr 10. PubMed PMID: 22496119.

[75]   Willcutt EG. The prevalence of DSM-IV attention-deficit/hyperactivity disorder: a
       meta-analytic review. *Neurotherapeutics.* 2012;9:490-9. doi: 10.1007/s13311-012-
       0135-8.

[76]   Payne JM, Hyman SL, Shores EA, North KN. Assessment of executive function and
       attention in children with neurofibromatosis type 1: relationships between cognitive
       measures and real-world behavior. *Child Neuropsychol.* 2011;17:313-29. doi:
       10.1080/09297049.2010.542746. PubMed PMID: 21347908.

[77]   Mautner VF, Granström S, Leark RA. .Impact of ADHD in Adults With
       Neurofibromatosis Type 1: Associated Psychological and Social Problems. *J Atten
       Disord.* 2012;10.

[78]   Brown JA, Emnett RJ, White CR, Yuede CM, Conyers SB, O'Malley KL, Wozniak DF,
       Gutmann DH. Reduced striatal dopamine underlies the attention system dysfunction in
       neurofibromatosis-1   mutant   mice.   *Hum   Mol   Genet.*   2010;19:4515-28.   doi:
       10.1093/hmg/ddq382.

[79]   Li W, Cui Y, Kushner SA, Brown RA, Jentsch JD, Frankland PW, Cannon TD, Silva
       AJ. The HMG-CoA reductase inhibitor lovastatin reverses the learning and attention
       deficits in a mouse model of neurofibromatosis type 1. *Curr Biol.* 2005;15:1961-7.

[80]   Chabernaud C, Mennes M, Kardel PG, Gaillard WD, Kalbfleisch ML, Vanmeter JW,
       Packer RJ, Milham MP, Castellanos FX, Acosta MT. Lovastatin regulates brain
       spontaneous low-frequency brain activity in neurofibromatosis type 1. *Neurosci Lett.*
       2012;515:28-33. doi: 10.1016/j.neulet.2012.03.009. Epub 2012 Mar 13.

[81]   Krab LC, de Goede-Bolder A, Aarsen FK, Pluijm SM, Bouman MJ, van der Geest JN,
       Lequin M, Catsman CE, Arts WF, Kushner SA, Silva AJ, de Zeeuw CI, Moll HA,
       Elgersma Y. Effect of simvastatin on cognitive functioning in children with
       neurofibromatosis type 1: a randomized controlled trial. *JAMA.* 2008;300:287-94. doi:
       10.1001/jama.300.3.287.

[82]   van der Vaart T, Plasschaert E, Rietman AB, Renard M, Oostenbrink R, Vogels A, de
       Wit MC, Descheemaeker MJ, Vergouwe Y, Catsman-Berrevoets CE, Legius E,
       Elgersma Y, Moll HA. Simvastatin for cognitive deficits and behavioural problems in
       patients with neurofibromatosis type 1 (NF1-SIMCODA): a randomised, placebo-
       controlled trial. *Lancet Neurol.* 2013;12:1076-83. doi: 10.1016/S1474-4422(13)70227-
       8. Epub 2013 Oct 1.

[83]   Aman MG, De Smedt G, Derivan A, Lyons B, Findling RL; Risperidone Disruptive
       Behavior Study Group. Double-blind, placebo-controlled study of risperidone for the
       treatment of disruptive behaviors in children with subaverage intelligence. *Am J
       Psychiatry.* 2002;159:1337-46.

[84]   Turgay A, Binder C, Snyder R, Fisman S. Long-term safety and efficacy of risperidone
       for the treatment of disruptive behavior disorders in children with subaverage IQs.
       Pediatrics. 2002;110:e34.

[85]   Aman MG, Binder C, Turgay A.Risperidone effects in the presence/absence of
       psychostimulant medicine in children with ADHD, other disruptive behavior disorders,
       and subaverage IQ. *J Child Adolesc Psychopharmacol. 2004*;14:243-54.

[86] Correia Filho AG, Bodanese R, Silva TL, Alvares JP, Aman M, Rohde LA.Comparison of risperidone and methylphenidate for reducing ADHD symptoms in children and adolescents with moderate mental retardation. *J Am Acad Child Adolesc Psychiatry.* 2005;44:748-55.

In: ADHD
Editors: Itai Berger and Adina Maeir

ISBN: 978-1-63321-047-9
© 2014 Nova Science Publishers, Inc.

Chapter 8

DSM-5, CONNECTIVITY AND NEUROPATHOLOGY: ADHD AND AUTISM AS AN EXAMPLE

Hanoch Cassuto, M.D., Ph.D.*

Pediatric Neurology Clinic, Leumit and Clalit HMO, Jersualem, Israel

ABSTRACT

Neurodevelopment is evolving into a multi-faceted field of scientific interest. Recent years have brought significant developments in the domain in both the research and the clinical point-of-view. The human brain mapping project, on the one hand, and the DSM-5 clinical manual, on the other, are two new developments that demonstrate this evolution. The progress of the science of neurodevelopment causes tension between these two domains, the neurobiological side tries to implement this science and the pathological derivatives under a scientific umbrella, measurement, while the clinical side tries to preserve the meaning behind the symptoms for efficient clinical work.

Autism Spectrum Disorder and Attention-Deficit-Hyperactivity Disorder are two classic examples that are researched intensively from each of these two approaches. In this article we will discuss the common issues as well as the controversial ones between clinical medical world and biological research.

INTRODUCTION

The medical world's attention has been recently focused on the newly released Diagnostic and Statistical Manual of Mental Disorders, Fifth Edition (DSM-5). Following previous editions footsteps, the new manual presents diagnostics of disorders and diseases that are primarily phenotypic and behavioral in nature. One of the main claims against this manual is that it is highly phenotypic and that today a more biological approach is required. Indeed, in the past two decades is enormous development in brain sciences. New tools, such as imaging, genetics and computerized methods have evolved, but still the causes of most

---

* Correspondence: Pediatric Neurology Clinic, Leumit and Clalit HMO, 17 A Diskin St, Jerusalem, Israel, 96440. E-mail: neuro.cog.c@gmail.com.

diseases in the manual remain obscure. The manual, which had also emerged into public awareness, is in the center of numerous debates and controversies. Time and extensive research will show which way the wind will blow.

One main topic of interest is Autism Spectrum Disorder (ASD). Beyond the changes in the definition of the disability and its leveling, the manual also addresses other controversies. Whereas autism was previously defined in the literature as a disability which encompasses other disabilities and cannot coexist with them, the new version of the DSM allows comorbidity with other disorders and diseases. One such comorbidity is Attention-Deficit/Hyperactivity Disorder (ADHD). Comorbidity is the simultaneous presence of two chronic diseases/conditions (whether or not independently) in a patient. In the past, ADHD and ASD were considered independent thus precluding co-occurrence of the disorders, leading to a long debate over the separation and treatment of both diagnoses. However, clinicians have long argued that both ASD and ADHD should be treated in parallel, and that an accurate evaluation should be done for each.

In the coming chapter I will deal with the ever developing science of the brain and the relations of the multi-domain brain networks to neurodevelopmental pathologies. I will discuss the proximities of ASD and ADHD to each other and the differences between the disorders and the accepted treatments for their comorbidity.

NETWORK BIOLOGY- A NEW CONCEPT

The last two decades are revolutionary in terms of data analysis. Supercomputers, advanced imaging and digitalization enabled science to deal with huge amounts of cumulative data and with these knowledge flourished. Biology was one particular science that evolved rapidly, and today we look with awe at biological systems that their understanding was only a dream or science fiction. All research levels are expanding, starting with structure in the macro scale to the microscopic details. The influence involves all of the biological domains-Physiology, Biochemistry, Genetics etc.

The ability to collect so many details and to analyze them, allowed scientists to read and decode data from different new sources. Imaging techniques, biological electrical currents and new ways of molecular dissection evolved to new "system biology". In that matter areas of great importance are the network sciences. Networks were known already for decades, their actual mathematics began in the 18th century, with the graph theory of Euler. It became important when computer sciences and networks became important in human life from the mid 20th century. The network way of thinking slowly permeated to the biological world, and its nomenclature became an integral part of scientific publications. Long standing questions find new, coherent answers according to the rules of these systems, and new solutions were given to some scientific mysteries.

Maybe the most important role of communication rule is the "small world" network. Science always learned through "regular" biological cascade or pathway, where one event causes the expected next one. Today, as we learned, most of the biological systems are much more complicated and events are connected and influenced by other events to create sophisticated networks [1]. There are centers that get the information and process it. The filtered information goes forward to the next center, higher in the hierarchy and so on.

Different network communicate with each other, to get in the end to the preferred response of the system (figure 1). These networks control, which is much more efficient than a regular system, enables better reaction flexibility, in a changing environment [2].

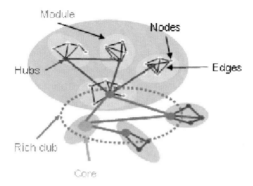

Figure 1. Hierarchic simple networks- nodes (grey) and edges create a module with a central node – called a hub (blue). The hubs in their turn create a new community – a "rich club" (red) which has a "core" (green) in its center.

THE BRAIN MAPPING

One of the areas most influenced by those methods is brain sciences [3]. In the beginning of the 20th century two scholars won the Nobel laoreal in Physiology or Medicine for their studies of the structure of the nervous system. Camillo Golgi together with Santiago Ramón y Cajal, received the Nobel Prize in 1906. A teacher and his colleague and former student were now in the middle of a scientific debate that changed neuroscience. The teacher (Golgi) believed in Gerlach theory - the Reticular Theory, which clamed that neurons form a diffuse network. His pupil, Cajal stated that the neurons are independent of one another, and are autonomous in their action. Cajal's Neuron Doctrine was widely accepted and actually the sole theory up to the end of the 20th century [4, 5]. Actually most of neuroscience was researched according to this theory, and the working hypothesis was of cascades of neuronal events. With the development of the network systems neurobiologists went "back to the future" and today it seems that both scholars were right. The reticulum of the brain is so complex, that both theories can live together. Surely any neuron has its own connection and acts as an individual, but the brain work can't be explained by a typical chain reaction. Today we know that the brain acts as "small world" networks. There are nodes and edges and hubs and rich clubs and core elements in each of those networks (Figure 2). In their turn they are working with other networks to be orchestrated by the changing needs of the organism. Some new insights relationship between networks helped us to better understand cognitive processes. For example one of the most researched networks communications is the task network versus the default network, in attention tasks [6, 7]. It was found that when an attention demanding task was given to a subject, some certain areas in the brain were marked positively in fMRI technique. When the same subject was resting another area lit up while the "task" area was not. It was also found that both areas were negatively coordinated. The "resting" area is called the "default system" which today plays an important role in attention research and understanding, and will be discussed later. The whole way of understanding the brain is by hierarchies of modules in the brain and their interactions. A whole new mapping system of the brain is replacing the former Brodmann's map (also from beginning of the 20th century) [8, 9]. Connectivity of the brain became a major target of research and understanding. Actually the importance of connectivity is so great that the US government funded human brain mapping project, as the next big scientific breakthrough after the genome project [10].

There are a lot of new tools enabling us to make the process. New techniques can analyze the structure of the brain from the macro scale [9] to the microscopic reticulum [11-13]. Those tools are using several variations of Magnetic Resonance Imaging (MRI)- volumetric, flow and functional. There are also measures that use more metabolic evaluations (as Positron Emission Tomography - PET) and some that measure electrical currents in the brain (as quantitative Electro Encephalo Gram - qEEG). All these tools are combined later on to create a whole new picture of the brain map [14].

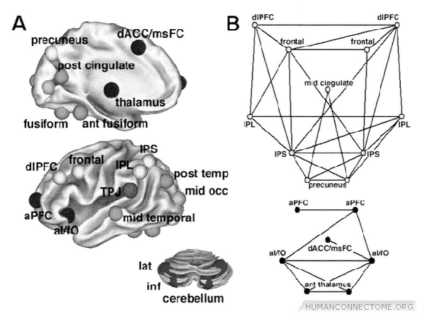

Figure 1. (A) Eight separate components that consitute a graph formed by regions involved in cognitive control, displayed on an inflated surface rendering of the brain. Nodes are color-doded according to separate components (or modules) of the control network. (B) Two-dimensional pseudoanatomical rendering of 2 components, the front-parietal component (yellow) and the cingulo-opercular component (black). (this picture was taken from the Human Connectome Project (funded by the National Institues of Health) http://www.humanconnectome.org/about/project/network-modeling.html).

HIERARCHY AND RELATIONS OF BRAIN NETWORKS

Today research revealed number of networks [for part of them- 8]. Some of them are more isolated in their function but others are communicating between themselves to create a complex system of reactions [15, 16]. The hierarchy of the network is complex and hubs in one network are nodes of the other (figure 1), up to the core network [17]. The sum of the process is not always clear and depends on what networks were dominating the message to the core area. This in turn can cause a different behavioral phenotype of the same disorder, depending on what network is less efficient, how high it is in the hierarchy and what is its role in a certain pathway.

The new maps of the brain are not only anatomical, but rather depend on relations and hierarchies of systems and their relations [18, 19]. The connections of systems can downsize, augment or inhibit connections of to other systems [for example- 20]. All these changes shift the focus on neuropathologies whether its "pure neurological" as epilepsy or "pure behavioral" as schizophrenia or neurodevelopmental as Attention deficit/hyperactivity disorder (ADHD), to become under one umbrella of research.

To add to the complexity, today the genetic networking (Genomics) and cortical maps [for example- 21], is major aspect in understanding the genetic milieu of pathological tendencies. The adding of this information helps to understand the developing of pathological conditions in the brain. With those tools, science today hope to give biological, maybe treatable, explanations to neuro-psychiatric pathologies in the future.

RELATION OF THE CLINICAL GUIDE (DSM-5) AND SCIENCE

With this evolution in the background *The Diagnostic and Statistical Manual of Mental Disorders* (5th ed.; DSM–5; American Psychiatric Association, 2013) which is the most widely accepted nomenclature used by clinicians and researchers for the classification of mental disorders, was published recently. The manual changed numerous diagnoses of former editions. The last DSM versions (DSM-IV and IV-R), were gradually becoming irrelevant because of the scientific "boom" of recent years. The new guide is trying to fill the gaps, and fit the era. There are more flexible definitions and more relation and place to biological background, even though that the manual remained clinical.

The best example for such a change in the manual is Autism Spectrum Disorder (ASD) which belongs to the new Neurodevelopmental section [22]. The definition was changed completely and is more flexible than it was with more specifiers [23]. This allows the clinician not only to give the diagnosis but to specify it with co-occurrence brain network pathologies. For example ASD with Rett's or Fragile-X syndromes (which are genetically defined disorders), or with epilepsy (which is neurological defined disease) or even to co-morbid with other DSM-5 defined and treatable disorders such as ADHD, Anxiety etc.

The flexibility of the symptoms gave the clinician more freedom to decide if the symptoms fit the general description. This approach sees the disorder as part of one spectrum and fit in to the understanding of networks and hierarchies. There is no need for segmentation of the disorder, but rather one disorder with different sequences and common end point. That is with understanding of the multifactorial genetic, epigenetic and environmental influences on the disorder. The main decision of the diagnostician is whether or not the individual crossed the threshold of this phenotypic disorder and to what extent (leveling).

Never the less, this is also the main weakness of the manual. Being too vague and changing too many definitions brought a lot of critique and the National Institute of Mental Health (NIMH), although accepted the DSM-5 as a clinical manual, did not accept it for research and research funding. For example, a quote from NIMH press release with the DSM-

5 publication [24] "…what may be realistically feasible today for practitioners is no longer sufficient for researchers…". A little earlier, another quote [25] "…That is why NIMH will be re-orienting its research away from DSM categories…". The Research Domain Criteria (RDoC) project of the NIMH is trying to change the "pure" clinical and sometime overlapping definitions of disorders to a more biological ground [26].

The new changes and definitions gave the notion of unstable "disorders". Phenotypic disorders can change according to the generation's state of mind, unlike biological defined diseases. This instability of diagnoses can undermine the reliability of the research, which was done according to the old definitions. For example, finding on brain connectivity of high functioning autistic subjects from the past is not reliable any more, especially if some of the subjects are not considered part of the spectrum and maybe not getting treatment that is needed [27, 28]. This can change the whole biological understanding that was built, and which one is the truth?

On the other hand, proponents claim that it's essential to research those phenotypic disorders with the new clinical definitions. Broadening them would include more brain circuits and can give the way to the understanding and help solving the biological questions of brain network and connectivity.

DSM-5 NEW APPROACH: ASD AND ADHD AS AN EXAMPLE

To demonstrate the new approach, the co-occurrence of ASD and ADHD would be discussed and whether or not they are on the same spectrum.

A major part of the network science is neurodevelopment. Today the importance of brain development is to such extent that even the first chapter in the psychiatric manual, the DSM-5, is called Neurodevelopmental Disorders [29]. The chapter combines numerous domains with inspiring new approach to these areas.

The neurodevelopmental research is blooming in all directions. Different age groups are being evaluated [30], and long term prospective studies are done [see- 31]. The categories are of normal developing groups [32], and groups of different types of neuropathology, with structural events as cerebral palsy [33], or of yet, unknown origin as ADHD, gray matter [34] or white matter [35]. Maybe the most researched group is the Attention deficit hyperactivity disorder. The research in of this wide spectrum disorder is expanding to several domains. Brain mapping of major attention connected areas are now available [8, 17], developmental changing area are being discovered [36]. Several disturbed or deficient networks were found [37, 38], and their response to medications was measured [38, 39].

The most recognized relationship between networks are between, the mentioned above, default system and task positive system with the salience network as a mediator [for review- 17]. In short, the default system is inhibited by the task-positive network in regular conditions allowing the subject to concentrate in the task he has to do. The default system kicks in when the person is "disconnected" from stimulation, external or internal. In ADHD this inhibition is not efficient and the default system interferes with the task positive network. Medicating the subject detach the networks and normalizes her abilities. This example is only one of those researched, and other networks are associated with the disorder [8].

Another neurodevelopmental disorder that is well investigated is Autistic Spectrum Disorder (ASD). The disabling morbidity and the rising incidence of the disorder are leading to wide and extensive research. For example in terms of genetic networks [see- 40] multi-gene processes are being explored. In terms of connectivity wide range research is done and the results show different brain areas that are involved in the disorder. [see- fMRI- 41; MEG- 42; qEEG- 43]. There is no use to enter the exact details of the revealed areas; some are under-connected [44], some are over-connected, and some are both [45].

It is interesting that an overlap was found between some of the clinical definitions, the genetic background and the symptoms of ADHD and ASD. If one looks at the phenotypic behavioral elements, that combine to diagnoses, there is some degree of overlap between them. Indeed, some of the most severely affected ADHD patients can be confusing for clinicians, with low social understanding and non communicational behaviors. This notion brought some researchers to refer the disorders as one spectrum [46, 47]. According to this claim actually there is a broad spectrum of the attention disorder, with autism at its end. This theory has a few obstacles some gene clusters are unique to autism [see- 40], and the networks and pathways that were mapped have some similarities but some major differences [48-50]. A possible explanation for the overlapping of both disorders is simple. The number of networks that exist is limited and it is not surprising that some end of pathological processes coincide. Moreover in the first DSM manuals autism was considered as part of childhood schizophrenia and indeed both pathologies share some similar symptoms. It is important to mention that ADHD response to some medical agents (with or without autism), while not changing the core symptoms of ASD. Even clinically, verbal working memory as an example- high functioning ASD children had different developmental trajectory than ADHD and their similar typically developing peers [51]

This chapter came after the end of a long debate. In the former DSM (DSM-IV), ADHD and autism couldn't co-occur. A diagnosis of pervasive developmental disorder of any kind ruled out other diagnoses including psychiatric as ADHD or syndromatic as Fragile X syndrome or even neurologic as epilepsy. The medical literature, especially in the last decade, referred to this approach as anachronistic. Extensive research and later reviews referred to autism as a disorder with comorbidities [see- 52, 53] and treated the patients for those co-occurrences as well [54]. Other comorbid psychopathologies also are diagnosed and treated with autism as depression, anxiety and aggressiveness [for review- 55]. The understanding that autism can co-occur with other illnesses, improved the treatment and life quality of the autistic patients. Even though the core symptoms weren't changed medically, treatment with medication to the accompanying disorders enabled the paramedical therapists to give better and more efficient therapy. The authors of the DSM-5 changed the definition of autism so it would fit the literature mood. Autism spectrum disorder changed in a lot of aspects- two core factors instead of three, leveling of the disorders [22] and as important enabling the clinician to diagnose a comorbid situation [23]. Actually the diagnosis of autism today demands specifiers and comorbidities as part of the later treatment plan. The clinician is expected to diagnose and differentiate between ASD symptoms and treatable ADHD symptoms. For example- does the inattention is primary, is it part of anxiety or it's simply lack of understanding the situation? Does the hyperactivity is because he "acts as if driven by a motor" or is it sensory seeking or sensory over responding?

An important addition to diagnosis, which can co-occur in both disorders, is the reaction to sensory input. This symptom re-entered the DSM-5 after being drawn out in the DSM-IV.

The term Sensory Processing Disorder (SPD) is a matter of debate [56, 57], and wasn't included in the current manual except in ASD. An accumulating data will help to differentiate the three categories (ASD, ADHD and SPD) and aim the treatment, and new publications help to find the difference between them [see- 58].

This debate is not the only one, and as the NIMH stated, there are no biological markers yet to the clinical disorders in the manual. The dissection of disorders, as was seen above is sometimes vague and some of the disorders are too pervasive or overlapping with others. The different spectrums can help to put the clinically defined population under one roof, but on the other hand they are multifactorial (Genetic, epigenetic and environmental) [59] and phenotypic. It is clear that in these conditions it would be hard to get to a single fitting mode of biological definition and treatment.

Another important dilemma is that even though the research is ongoing for two decades at least it's still preliminary. The imaging and electrical research are mainly statistical, and depend on cooperation the participants. Recently an interesting research was published and challenged all tracts that were found to be disturbed in autism except one [60]. This diffusion-weighted imaging research found at first all the tracts that were found in the past. After controlling for head motion all these effects disappear and only one tract remained as a sole different from controls. When dealing with participants that can be hyperactive, anxious or sensory overwhelmed it is clear that this option should be considered. Even more then that a bias of research is obvious, because subjects have to be high functioning to complete tasks in fMRI and the results that are published relate only to this population.

CONCLUSION

The brain mapping project is just starting out and awareness to the difficulties will improve the results and tapering of biases as mentioned. It seem today that the brain network and their relation that some are mutual to different disorders and some are unique, would create new nomenclature that is more accurate and more biological defined. Already new segmentation of the population arise [48] with ASD with or without ADHD and their distinct brain appearance. This in turn will help the clinician to target their treatment.

The DSM-5 manual is enabling today both the diagnosis of autism and the comorbidities. The clinician today can treat the later and improve the patient quality of life and availability for therapies. The future treatment could be aimed not only for psychiatric or neurological illnesses, but also to etiologies as Fragile-X or Rett syndromes [61]. We also hope that we could even treat core symptoms with the extensively growing knowledge.

REFERENCES

[1]   Bullmore E, Sporns O. The economy of brain network organization. *Nat Rev Neurosci.* 2012 Apr 13;13(5):336-49. doi: 10.1038/nrn3214.

[2]   Morgan JL, Lichtman JW. Why not connectomics? *Nat Methods.* 2013 Jun;10(6):494-500. doi: 10.1038/nmeth.2480. PubMed PMID: 23722208.

[3] Sporns O. Making sense of brain network data. *Nat Methods.* 2013 Jun;10(6):491-3. doi: 10.1038/nmeth.2485. PubMed PMID: 23722207.

[4] Bock O. Cajal, Golgi, Nansen, Schäfer and the neuron doctrine. *Endeavour.* 2013 Dec;37(4):228-34. doi: 10.1016/j.endeavour.2013.06.006. Epub 2013 Jul 17. PubMed PMID: 23870749.

[5] Sotelo C. Camillo Golgi and Santiago Ramon y Cajal: the anatomical organization of the cortex of the cerebellum. Can the neuron doctrine still support our actual knowledge on the cerebellar structural arrangement? *Brain Res Rev.* 2011 Jan 7;66(1-2):16-34. doi: 10.1016/j.brainresrev.2010.05.004. Epub 2010 May 26. PubMed PMID: 20621648.

[6] Kelly AM, Uddin LQ, Biswal BB, Castellanos FX, Milham MP. Competition between functional brain networks mediates behavioral variability. *Neuroimage.* 2008 Jan 1;39(1):527-37. Epub 2007 Aug 23. PubMed PMID: 17919929.

[7] Fox MD, Snyder AZ, Vincent JL, Corbetta M, Van Essen DC, Raichle ME. The human brain is intrinsically organized into dynamic, anticorrelated functional networks. *Proc Natl Acad Sci U S A.* 2005 Jul 5;102(27):9673-8. Epub 2005 Jun 23. PubMed PMID: 15976020; PubMed Central PMCID: PMC1157105.

[8] Whitfield-Gabrieli S, Ford JM. Default mode network activity and connectivity in psychopathology. *Annu Rev Clin Psychol.* 2012;8:49-76. doi: 10.1146/annurev-clinpsy-032511-143049. Epub 2012 Jan 6. Review. PubMed PMID: 22224834.

[9] Craddock RC, Jbabdi S, Yan CG, Vogelstein JT, Castellanos FX, Di Martino A, Kelly C, Heberlein K, Colcombe S, Milham MP. *Imaging human connectomes at the macroscale. Nat Methods.* 2013 Jun;10(6):524-39. doi: 10.1038/nmeth.2482. PubMed PMID: 23722212.

[10] *Fact Sheet: BRAIN Initiative,* 2013, http://www.whitehouse.gov/the-press-office/2013/04/02/ fact-sheet-brain-initiative

[11] Osten P, Margrie TW. Mapping brain circuitry with a light microscope. *Nat Methods.* 2013 Jun;10(6):515-23. doi: 10.1038/nmeth.2477. Review. PubMed PMID: 23722211.

[12] Cai D, Cohen KB, Luo T, Lichtman JW, Sanes JR. Improved tools for the Brainbow toolbox. Nat Methods. 2013 Jun;10(6):540-7. PubMed PMID: 23866336.

[13] Chung K, Deisseroth K. CLARITY for mapping the nervous system. Nat Methods. 2013 Jun;10(6):508-13. doi: 10.1038/nmeth.2481. Erratum in: *Nat Methods.* 2013 Oct;10(10):1035. PubMed PMID: 23722210.

[14] Sporns O. The human connectome: a complex network. *Ann N Y Acad Sci.* 2011 Apr;1224:109-25. doi: 10.1111/j.1749-6632.2010.05888.x. Epub 2011 Jan 4. PubMed PMID: 21251014.

[15] Sepulcre J, Sabuncu MR, Yeo TB, Liu H, Johnson KA. Stepwise connectivity of the modal cortex reveals the multimodal organization of the human brain. *J Neurosci.* 2012 Aug 1;32(31):10649-61. PubMed PMID: 22855814; PubMed Central PMCID: PMC3483645.

[16] van den Heuvel MP, Sporns O. Network hubs in the human brain. *Trends Cogn Sci.* 2013 Dec;17(12):683-96. doi: 10.1016/j.tics.2013.09.012. PubMed PMID: 24231140.

[17] Castellanos FX, Proal E. Large-scale brain systems in ADHD: beyond the prefrontal-striatal model. Trends Cogn Sci. 2012 Jan;16(1):17-26. doi:10.1016/j.tics.2011.11.007. Epub 2011 Dec 12. Review. PubMed PMID: 22169776; PubMed Central PMCID: PMC3272832.

[18] Catani M, Dell'acqua F, Vergani F, Malik F, Hodge H, Roy P, Valabregue R, Thiebaut de Schotten M. Short frontal lobe connections of the human brain. *Cortex.* 2012 Feb;48(2):273-91. doi: 10.1016/j.cortex.2011.12.001. Epub 2011 Dec 13. PubMed PMID: 22209688.

[19] Bressler SL, Menon V. Large-scale brain networks in cognition: emerging methods and principles. *Trends Cogn Sci.* 2010 Jun;14(6):277-90. doi:10.1016/j.tics.2010.04.004. Epub 2010 May 20. Review. PubMed PMID: 20493761.

[20] Forster S, Nunez Elizalde AO, Castle E, Bishop SJ. Unraveling the Anxious Mind: Anxiety, Worry, and Frontal Engagement in Sustained Attention Versus Off-Task Processing. *Cereb Cortex.* 2013 Sep 22. [Epub ahead of print] PubMed PMID: 24062316.

[21] Chen CH, Gutierrez ED, Thompson W, Panizzon MS, Jernigan TL, Eyler LT, Fennema-Notestine C, Jak AJ, Neale MC, Franz CE, Lyons MJ, Grant MD, Fischl B, Seidman LJ, Tsuang MT, Kremen WS, Dale AM. Hierarchical genetic organization of human cortical surface area. *Science.* 2012 Mar 30;335(6076):1634-6. doi: 10.1126/science.1215330. PubMed PMID: 22461613; PubMed Central PMCID: PMC3690329.

[22] American Psychiatric Association. (2013). *Diagnostic and statistical manual of mental disorders (5th ed.).* Arlington, VA: American Psychiatric Publishing. Pps. 50-59 (American Psychiatric Association, 2013).

[23] Grzadzinski R, Huerta M, Lord C. DSM-5 and autism spectrum disorders (ASDs): an opportunity for identifying ASD subtypes. *Mol Autism.* 2013 May 15;4(1):12. doi: 10.1186/2040-2392-4-12. PubMed PMID: 23675638; PubMed Central PMCID: PMC3671160.

[24] DSM-5 and RDoC: Shared Interests May 13, 2013, http://www.nimh.nih.gov/news/ science-news/2013/dsm-5-and-rdoc-shared-interests.shtml

[25] Thomas Insel on April 29, 2013, in http://www.nimh.nih.gov/about/director/2013/ transforming-diagnosis.shtml

[26] Casey BJ, Craddock N, Cuthbert BN, Hyman SE, Lee FS, Ressler KJ. DSM-5 and RDoC: progress in psychiatry research? *Nat Rev Neurosci.* 2013 Nov;14(11):810-4. doi: 10.1038/nrn3621. Review. PubMed PMID: 24135697.

[27] Matson JL, Hattier MA, Williams LW. How does relaxing the algorithm for autism affect DSM-V prevalence rates? *J Autism Dev Disord.* 2012 Aug;42(8):1549-56. doi: 10.1007/s10803-012-1582-0. PubMed PMID: 22733300.

[28] Beighley JS, Matson JL, Rieske RD, Jang J, Cervantes PE, Goldin RL. *Comparing challenging behavior in children diagnosed with autism spectrum disorders according to the DSM-IV-TR and the proposed DSM-5. Dev Neurorehabil.* 2013 Dec;16(6):375-81. doi: 10.3109/17518423.2012.760119. Epub 2013 Mar 11. PubMed PMID: 23477536.

[29] American Psychiatric Association. (2013). *Diagnostic and statistical manual of mental disorders* (5th ed.). Arlington, VA: American Psychiatric Publishing. Pps. 30-86 (American Psychiatric Association, 2013).

[30] Gong G, Rosa-Neto P, Carbonell F, Chen ZJ, He Y, Evans AC. Age- and gender-related differences in the cortical anatomical network. *J Neurosci.* 2009 Dec 16;29(50):15684-93. doi: 10.1523/JNEUROSCI.2308-09.2009. PubMed PMID: 20016083; PubMed Central PMCID: PMC2831804.

[31]   Lebel C, Beaulieu C. Longitudinal development of human brain wiring continues from childhood into adulthood. *J Neurosci.* 2011 Jul 27;31(30):10937-47. doi:10.1523/JNEUROSCI.5302-10.2011. PubMed PMID: 21795544.

[32]   Dennis EL, Thompson PM. Mapping connectivity in the developing brain. *Int J Dev Neurosci.* 2013 Nov;31(7):525-42. doi: 10.1016/j.ijdevneu.2013.05.007. Epub 2013 May 27. PubMed PMID: 23722009; PubMed Central PMCID: PMC3800504.

[33]   Englander ZA, Pizoli CE, Batrachenko A, Sun J, Worley G, Mikati MA, Kurtzberg J, Song AW. Diffuse reduction of white matter connectivity in cerebral palsy with specific vulnerability of long range fiber tracts. *Neuroimage Clin.* 2013 Mar 22;2:440-7. doi: 10.1016/j.nicl.2013.03.006. eCollection 2013. PubMed PMID: 24179798; PubMed Central PMCID: PMC3777769.

[34]   Proal E, Reiss PT, Klein RG, Mannuzza S, Gotimer K, Ramos-Olazagasti MA, Lerch JP, He Y, Zijdenbos A, Kelly C, Milham MP, Castellanos FX. Brain gray matter deficits at 33-year follow-up in adults with attention-deficit/hyperactivity disorder established in childhood. *Arch Gen Psychiatry.* 2011 Nov;68(11):1122-34. doi: 10.1001/ archgenpsychiatry.2011.117. PubMed PMID: 22065528; PubMed Central PMCID: PMC3554238.

[35]   Cortese S, Imperati D, Zhou J, Proal E, Klein RG, Mannuzza S, Ramos-Olazagasti MA, Milham MP, Kelly C, Castellanos FX. White matter alterations at 33-year follow-up in adults with childhood attention-deficit/hyperactivity disorder. *Biol Psychiatry.* 2013 Oct 15;74(8):591-8. doi:10.1016/j.biopsych.2013.02.025. Epub 2013 Apr 6. PubMed PMID: 23566821; PubMed Central PMCID: PMC3720804.

[36]   Shaw P, Malek M, Watson B, Sharp W, Evans A, Greenstein D. Development of cortical surface area and gyrification in attention-deficit/hyperactivity disorder. *Biol Psychiatry.* 2012 Aug 1;72(3):191-7. doi:10.1016/j.biopsych.2012.01.031. Epub 2012 Mar 13. PubMed PMID: 22418014.

[37]   Noreika V, Falter CM, Rubia K. Timing deficits in attention-deficit/hyperactivity disorder (ADHD): *evidence from neurocognitive and neuroimaging studies. Neuropsychologia.* 2013 Jan;51(2):235-66. doi:10.1016/j.neuropsychologia. 2012.09.036. Epub 2012 Sep 28. Review. PubMed PMID:23022430.

[38]   Nakao T, Radua J, Rubia K, Mataix-Cols D. Gray matter volume abnormalities in ADHD: voxel-based meta-analysis exploring the effects of age and stimulant medication. *Am J Psychiatry.* 2011 Nov;168(11):1154-63. doi:10.1176/appi.ajp. 2011.11020281. Epub 2011 Aug 24. PubMed PMID: 21865529.

[39]   Cubillo A, Smith AB, Barrett N, Giampietro V, Brammer MJ, Simmons A, Rubia K. Shared and drug-specific effects of atomoxetine and methylphenidate on inhibitory brain dysfunction in medication-naive ADHD boys. *Cereb Cortex.* 2014 Jan;24(1):174-85. doi: 10.1093/cercor/bhs296. Epub 2012 Oct 9. PubMed PMID: 23048018; PubMed Central PMCID: PMC3862268.

[40]   Ben-David E, Shifman S. Networks of neuronal genes affected by common and rare variants in autism spectrum disorders. *PLoS Genet.* 2012;8(3):e1002556. doi:10.1371/ journal.pgen.1002556. Epub 2012 Mar 8. PubMed PMID: 22412387; PubMed Central PMCID: PMC3297570.

[41]   Rudie JD, Shehzad Z, Hernandez LM, Colich NL, Bookheimer SY, Iacoboni M, Dapretto M. Reduced functional integration and segregation of distributed neural systems underlying social and emotional information processing in autism spectrum

disorders. *Cereb Cortex.* 2012 May;22(5):1025-37. doi:10.1093/cercor/bhr171. Epub 2011 Jul 22. PubMed PMID: 21784971; PubMed Central PMCID: PMC3328339

[42]   Kikuchi M, Shitamichi K, Yoshimura Y, Ueno S, Hiraishi H, Hirosawa T, Munesue T, Nakatani H, Tsubokawa T, Haruta Y, Oi M, Niida Y, Remijn GB, Takahashi T, Suzuki M, Higashida H, Minabe Y. Altered brain connectivity in 3-to 7-year-old children with autism spectrum disorder. *Neuroimage Clin.* 2013 Mar 19;2:394-401. doi: 10.1016/j.nicl.2013.03.003. eCollection 2013. PubMed PMID: 24179793; PubMed Central PMCID: PMC3777701.

[43]   Barttfeld P, Amoruso L, Ais J, Cukier S, Bavassi L, Tomio A, Manes F, Ibanez A, Sigman M. Organization of brain networks governed by long-range connections index autistic traits in the general population. *J Neurodev Disord.* 2013 Jun 27;5(1):16. doi: 10.1186/1866-1955-5-16. PubMed PMID: 23806204; PubMed Central PMCID: PMC3698083.

[44]   Uddin LQ, Menon V. The anterior insula in autism: under-connected and under-examined. *Neurosci Biobehav Rev.* 2009 Sep;33(8):1198-203. doi:10.1016/ j.neubiorev.2009.06.002. Epub 2009 Jun 16. Review. PubMed PMID: 19538989; PubMed Central PMCID: PMC2743776.

[45]   Markram K, Markram H. The intense world theory - a unifying theory of the neurobiology of autism. *Front Hum Neurosci.* 2010 Dec 21;4:224. doi:10.3389/fnhum.2010.00224. eCollection 2010. PubMed PMID: 21191475; PubMed Central PMCID: PMC3010743.

[46]   Rommelse NN, Franke B, Geurts HM, Hartman CA, Buitelaar JK. Shared heritability of attention-deficit/hyperactivity disorder and autism spectrum disorder. *Eur Child Adolesc Psychiatry.* 2010 Mar;19(3):281-95. doi:10.1007/s00787-010-0092-x. Epub 2010 Feb 11. Review. PubMed PMID: 20148275; PubMed Central PMCID: PMC2839489.

[47]   Rommelse NN, Geurts HM, Franke B, Buitelaar JK, Hartman CA. A review on cognitive and brain endophenotypes that may be common in autism spectrum disorder and attention-deficit/hyperactivity disorder and facilitate the search for pleiotropic genes. *Neurosci Biobehav Rev.* 2011 May;35(6):1363-96. doi:10.1016/j.neubiorev. 2011.02.015. Epub 2011 Mar 4. Review. PubMed PMID: 21382410.

[48]   Di Martino A, Zuo XN, Kelly C, Grzadzinski R, Mennes M, Schvarcz A, Rodman J, Lord C, Castellanos FX, Milham MP. Shared and distinct intrinsic functional network centrality in autism and attention-deficit/hyperactivity disorder. *Biol Psychiatry.* 2013 Oct 15;74(8):623-32. doi: 10.1016/j.biopsych.2013.02.011. Epub 2013 Mar 28. PubMed PMID: 23541632.

[49]   Christakou A, Murphy CM, Chantiluke K, Cubillo AI, Smith AB, Giampietro V, Daly E, Ecker C, Robertson D; MRC AIMS consortium, Murphy DG, Rubia K. Disorder-specific functional abnormalities during sustained attention in youth with Attention Deficit Hyperactivity Disorder (ADHD) and with autism. *Mol Psychiatry.* 2013 Feb;18(2):236-44. doi: 10.1038/mp.2011.185. Epub 2012 Jan 31. Erratum in: Mol Psychiatry. 2013 Feb;18(2):264. PubMed PMID: 22290121; PubMed Central PMCID: PMC3554878.

[50]   Lim L, Marquand A, Cubillo AA, Smith AB, Chantiluke K, Simmons A, Mehta M, Rubia K. Disorder-specific predictive classification of adolescents with attention deficit hyperactivity disorder (ADHD) relative to autism using structural magnetic resonance

imaging. *PLoS One.* 2013 May 16;8(5):e63660. doi:10.1371/journal.pone.0063660. Print 2013. PubMed PMID: 23696841; PubMed Central PMCID: PMC3656087.

[51] Andersen PN, Skogli EW, Hovik KT, Geurts H, Egeland J, Oie M. Working memory arrest in children with high-functioning autism compared to children with attention-deficit/hyperactivity disorder: Results from a 2-year longitudinal study. *Autism.* 2014 Mar 6. [Epub ahead of print] PubMed PMID: 24604922.

[52] Gargaro BA, Rinehart NJ, Bradshaw JL, Tonge BJ, Sheppard DM. Autism and ADHD: how far have we come in the comorbidity debate? *Neurosci Biobehav Rev.* 2011 Apr;35(5):1081-8. doi: 10.1016/j.neubiorev.2010.11.002. Epub 2010 Nov 18. PubMed PMID: 21093480.

[53] Matson JL, Rieske RD, Williams LW. The relationship between autism spectrum disorders and attention-deficit/hyperactivity disorder: an overview. *Res Dev Disabil.* 2013 Sep;34(9):2475-84. doi: 10.1016/j.ridd.2013.05.021. Epub 2013 Jun 7. PubMed PMID: 23751293.

[54] Davis NO, Kollins SH. Treatment for co-occurring attention deficit/hyperactivity disorder and autism spectrum disorder. *Neurotherapeutics.* 2012 Jul;9(3):518-30. doi: 10.1007/s13311-012-0126-9. Review. PubMed PMID:22678458; PubMed Central PMCID: PMC3441928.

[55] Matson JL, Cervantes PE. Commonly studied comorbid psychopathologies among persons with autism spectrum disorder. *Res Dev Disabil.* 2014 Mar 11. pii:S0891-4222(14)00080-8. doi: 10.1016/j.ridd.2014.02.012. [Epub ahead of print]. PubMed PMID: 24629541.

[56] Section On Complementary And Integrative Medicine; Council on Children with Disabilities; American Academy of Pediatrics, Zimmer M, Desch L. Sensory integration therapies for children with developmental and behavioral disorders. *Pediatrics.* 2012 Jun;129(6):1186-9. doi: 10.1542/peds.2012-0876. Epub 2012 May 28. PubMed PMID: 22641765.

[57] *Letter to the Editor Re: Sensory Integration Therapies for Children with Developmental and behavioral Disorders* Miller LJ 2012, http:// pediatrics.aappublications.org/content/ 129/6/1186.long/reply#pediatrics_el_53841

[58] Owen JP, Marco EJ, Desai S, Fourie E, Harris J, Hill SS, Arnett AB, Mukherjee P. Abnormal white matter microstructure in children with sensory processing disorders. *Neuroimage Clin.* 2013 Jun 23;2:844-53. doi:10.1016/j.nicl.2013.06.009. eCollection 2013. PubMed PMID: 24179836; PubMed Central PMCID: PMC3778265.

[59] Geschwind DH. Genetics of autism spectrum disorders. *Trends Cogn Sci.* 2011 Sep;15(9):409-16. doi: 10.1016/j.tics.2011.07.003. Epub 2011 Aug 18. PubMed PMID: 21855394; PubMed Central PMCID: PMC3691066.

[60] Koldewyn K, Yendiki A, Weigelt S, Gweon H, Julian J, Richardson H, Malloy C, Saxe R, Fischl B, Kanwisher N. Differences in the right inferior longitudinal fasciculus but no general disruption of white matter tracts in children with autism spectrum disorder. *Proc Natl Acad Sci U S A.* 2014 Feb 4;111(5):1981-6. doi: 10.1073/pnas.1324037111. Epub 2014 Jan 21. PubMed PMID: 24449864; PubMed Central PMCID: PMC3918797.

[61] Picker JD, Walsh CA. New innovations: therapeutic opportunities for intellectual disabilities. *Ann Neurol.* 2013 Sep;74(3):382-90. doi:10.1002/ana.24002. Review. PubMed PMID: 24038210; PubMed Central PMCID:PMC3876407.

In: ADHD
Editors: Itai Berger and Adina Maeir

ISBN: 978-1-63321-047-9
© 2014 Nova Science Publishers, Inc.

Chapter 9

ATTENTION DEFICIT HYPERACTIVITY DISORDER AMONG CHILDREN WITH CHRONIC DISEASES

Itai Berger, M.D.*

Director of the Neuro-Cognitive Center, Division of Pediatrics,
Hadassah-Hebrew University Medical Center, Jerusalem, Israel

ABSTRACT

There is a correlation between children's health condition, the existence of chronic disease and the cognitive and academic performance. It was observed for many years that different chronic health conditions predispose children to different kinds of neuro-cognitive impairments, including – lower cognitive level, learning disabilities, behavioral difficulties and ADHD. But, the characteristics of impaired performance or ability secondary to poor health are commonly not understood. In order to prevent, correctly diagnose and improve neuro-cognitive performance among children with chronic illness, there is a need to clarify and quantify the relationship between a variety of chronic health conditions and children's cognitive performance and ability. This chapter summarizes what is known through published research about the association of cognitive performance, especially attention abilities with chronic health conditions such as diabetes mellitus, seizure disorders, asthma, chronic kidney disease, and other chronic conditions. Better understanding of those important factors and relations will hopefully result in information that will help us understand how to reduce the impact of chronic disease on cognitive function, school performance, and quality of life in children and adolescents.

INTRODUCTION

Chronic medical conditions seriously impair long term health and cognitive function in the pediatric population [1]. Over the past years, there is an improvement in health care delivered to children and youth with special medical needs due to improved identification and

---

* Correspondence: Itai Berger, M.D., The Neuro-Cognitive Center, Hadassah-Hebrew University Medical Center, POB 24035, Mount Scopus, Jerusalem, Israel, 91240. E-mail: itberg@hadassah.org.il.

classification of disabling conditions, new medical interventions, and the promotion of school and community inclusion programs. Such interventions can increase opportunities for these children in the adult world with increased educational, work, and recreational supports and inclusionary programs. Many efforts are directed for preventing those with a chronic illness or disability to experience condition related disparities [2].

ADHD is a manageable, chronic condition that frequently persists into adulthood. It is one of the most common chronic conditions of childhood [3]. ADHD is in fact the most prevalent neuro-developmental disorder among children. In the United States, approximately 5.4 million children between 6 and 17 years of age (9.5% of all U.S. children) have received an ADHD diagnosis [4]. Like other chronic health conditions, ADHD is more severe in lower socioeconomic groups, is usually treated in the primary care setting and demonstrates symptoms that often persist into adulthood [5]. ADHD is associated with low rates of high-school graduation and completion of postsecondary education and poor peer-relationships, even when it is appropriately managed, leading to high economic and social burdens [6]. Compared with some other chronic health conditions, children and adolescents with ADHD use more health care money and may be less adherent to treatment plans [3, 7].

Much work has been done to improve the quality of primary care for children and adolescents with chronic disorders [2], but not enough is known about the connection between chronic health conditions and cognitive performance such as attention deficits.

Since we suspect that among children with chronic health conditions there is lower recognition of and treatment levels for ADHD, any approach promoting and improving early and accurate diagnosis and treatment as well as disparity prevention must take into account the overlap of ADHD existence among children with chronic health conditions [8]. Efforts to improve quality of care, diagnosis and treatment for youth with ADHD in the context of improving overall care of chronic conditions will likely have positive effects [3]. Primary care clinicians are likely to spend more time learning about the family's cultural beliefs, approaches to chronic health condition and disability, understanding, and expectations [9]. These clinicians are more likely to provide parents with education materials in the appropriate language and with appropriate cultural understanding. They may also be more likely to identify and address the socioeconomic and cultural barriers (such as transportation obstacles, inconvenient hours for health care visits, or cultural beliefs and community customs) that influence the child's health and well-being [2]. This chapter illuminates these serious and persistent problems and provides a stimulus to approach ADHD among children and adolescents with other chronic conditions. The efforts to do so are worthy of many of the changes made in health care delivery to improve comprehensive care for patients with chronic conditions. Specifically, we focus on how a comprehensive approach to ADHD as a chronic disorder could improve quality of life and long term complications and to develop strategies that will help to overcome barriers and disparities among children with the common overlap of ADHD and other chronic health condition.

GENERAL CONCEPTS

To regulate and guide behavior through a constantly changing environment, the brain requires a central coordinating system. The executive system (ES) is responsible for the simultaneous operation of a number of cognitive processes in charge of goal-directed, task-oriented behaviors, self-regulation and behavior inhibition as well as planning, working memory, mental flexibility, response inhibition, impulse control and monitoring of action [10]. Any dysfunction of the ES affects the child's executive functions (EF) impairing his/her ability to analyze, plan, prioritize, schedule, initiate and complete an activity in a timely manner [11]. Attention deficit hyperactivity disorder (ADHD) is an early onset, clinically heterogeneous, complex neurobiological disorder, defined by persistent symptoms of inattention and hyperactivity/impulsivity that cause impairment in two or more settings according to DSM-5 [12]. It has been associated with a broad range of impairments for those affected, including (but not limited to) cognitive, academic, behavioral, emotional and social functioning. Additionally, ADHD in children and adolescents is frequently associated with comorbidities, including learning disabilities, mood disorders, conduct disorder, oppositional defiant disorders, anxiety disorders and substance use disorders [13]. The pathophysiology of ADHD is marked by dopaminergic and nonadrenergic dysregulation, as well as by structural and functional abnormalities of the cortico-cortical and fronto-subcortical pathways, including those of the striatum and cerebellum. Children with ADHD have serious difficulties with EF in so many areas that some psychiatrists and psychologists have proposed renaming this disorder as EF disorder or EF deficit disorder [14]. Many of the executive dysfunctions are found in children with ADHD including difficulties with priority and time management, planning and organization, initiating and completing tasks in a timely manner, difficulty shifting cognitive set, a high level of procrastination, forgetfulness and poor working memory [11]. Managing time and meeting deadlines then become a huge problem. These children need constant reminders because of problems with working memory. They are unable to change behaviors or plans according to environmental demands and have difficulties reconfiguring an alternate plan when presented with new situations or tasks. They live mainly in the here and now, do not deal with contradictions well and cannot adapt to changes or changing situations quickly. They do not shift easily, can get stuck on one routine, hyper-focus on one task and are rigid in their thinking. In their social interactions they expect their peers as well as parents to behave in predictable ways and when this does not happen they try to control the situation, react excessively or go to a shutdown mode [15].

The prefrontal cortex (PFC) is a highly evolved cortical area that is essential for regulating attention, cognitive control, motivation, and emotion. Distinct regions of PFC regulate this spectrum of functions, with the dorsolateral PFC (DLPFC) regulating attention, planning, and working memory, and the inferior frontal cortex (IFC) mediating functions of cognitive control such as inhibitory control, interference control, and cognitive flexibility. The lateral orbitofrontal (OFC) and the ventromedial PFC (including orbital) (VMPFC) regulate emotion and motivation. The anterior cingulate cortex, which many consider to be a PFC sub-region, is similarly organized such that the most caudal region regulates movement, more anterior regions regulate attention/cognition, and the most rostral and ventral regions regulate emotion and motivation. Top-down regulation by the PFC arises from its extensive connections to posterior cortical and subcortical structures, including parallel circuits through the basal ganglia and cerebellum specialized for each processing domain [16].

Neuroimaging studies in patients with ADHD have shown consistent deficits in structure and function as well as interregional structural and functional connectivity in the IFC and DLPFC circuitries that mediate attention and inhibitory control, with the most prominent structural deficits in the basal ganglia. Furthermore, longitudinal imaging studies show that the impairment in these late developing DLPFC and IFC fronto-striato-cerebellar and fronto-parietal systems may be due to a late structural cortical maturation [13, 16, 17].

Given the wide heterogeneity and complex manifestations of ADHD, recent theoretical work has suggested the importance of a developmental perspective that views ADHD as a multi-factorial disorder with multiple, causal processes, and pathways through development [18]. The developmental psychopathology perspective attempts to specify the developmental pathways that are associated with ADHD and to predict outcome of the disorder, by looking at the interaction of genetic and environmental risk factors. The etiology of ADHD thus points toward risk factors that operate very early in life. This is consistent with clinical and epidemiological data suggesting an early onset of ADHD symptoms [19]. The speed of maturation of the central nervous system (CNS) can be modified under the influence of the environment. From fertilization biological maturing processes are continuously at work. These processes depend on individual experience within a given environment, the constraints of that environment, and the educational attitudes of the people surrounding the child. The most dramatic brain developmental changes occur during the first years of life. Therefore, damage to CNS during this critical developmental period can lead to persistent neurocognitive impairments [19].

There is a correlation between children's general health and cognitive performance. That generalization is not often accompanied by a discussion of specific health conditions or factors and more rarely accompanied by evidence. Moreover, the characteristics of impaired performance or ability secondary to poor health are commonly not understood. Since ADHD is the most common neuro-developmental disorder of childhood and is among the most prevalent chronic health conditions affecting school-age children, than we assume that if chronic disorders in childhood have are major influential factor regarding cognitive and behavioral processes, it should have an effect on the development of ADHD in children [12, 13]. It is possible to hypothesize that since chronic health conditions affect brain performance less brain reserve capacity serves as a vulnerability factor for subsequent brain dysfunction. As an example, were one to compare two individuals, one with a higher cognitive reserve, and one with a lower reserve, both of whom now experience the same brain insult, that individual with less reserve will show greater cognitive deterioration. The association of ADHD and attention performance with other chronic diseases is not so well studied [20].

This chapter summarizes what is known through published research about the association of ADHD with common diseases and conditions affecting children.

DIABETES MELLITUS (DM)

Children with diabetes have a shortage of insulin or a decreased ability to use insulin, a hormone that allows glucose to enter cells and be converted to energy. There are two main types of diabetes. Type 1 most often appears during childhood or adolescence. Type 2 diabetes, which is linked to obesity and physical inactivity, accounts for 90% to 95% of diabetes cases and most often appears among people older than 40 years. With the onset of the obesity epidemic, however, type 2 is being diagnosed in higher numbers of children and teenagers. In addition to the recent and publicized increase in type 2 diabetes among youth, the incidence of childhood type-1 diabetes also has increased [20]. Treatment of DM requires multiple daily injections of insulin. Complications of the disease include hypoglycemia and hyperglycemia, which can have an impact on children's attention performance [21]. Most published studies about diabetes and cognitive performance among children, demonstrate an association between poor cognitive functioning and early onset of diabetes (younger than 5 years) and/or a history of severe hypoglycemic episodes [22]. The specific nature of the deficit varies, but verbal IQ, visuo-spatial/nonverbal functioning, memory, and attention have all shown to be affected.

Despite differing research methods, there appears to be an emerging consensus from the data, which is that children with diabetes are more likely to be at a cognitive and academic disadvantage. The existence and magnitude of this disadvantage is related to early onset diabetes and severe fluctuations in metabolic control, especially if the child experienced seizures, unconsciousness, or ketoacidosis as result of the poor control. Boys appear to be at a relatively greater risk for learning problems than girls. Of these 2 risk factors, only the second factor (prevention of wide fluctuations in glucose control) can be influenced by school policies and practices. The relevance of good glucose control to long-term and short-term health as well as to academic functioning should serve to make the support of using these technologies in school more compelling for educational reasons. Theoretically, the association between better control and academic functioning can be an incentive to public and private educational systems and their professionals and staff to provide assistance and support to students with diabetes who require help with pump therapy, close observation for signs of hypoglycemia, and rapid responses by staff members trained to respond to severe hypoglycemic episodes [20].

EPILEPSY

ADHD and epilepsy are both common childhood disorders and both can have significant negative consequences on a child's behavioral, learning, and social development. Both conditions can co-occur and population studies suggest that the prevalence of ADHD in childhood epilepsy is between 12 and 17%. The prevalence of epilepsy in ADHD is lower but it is not clear if the rate of epilepsy is higher in ADHD populations than in the general population [23]. The difficulties with describing the direct effect of epilepsy on cognitive, academic, attentional, and school performance are that epilepsy is highly linked to other conditions that affect school functioning (seizures occur in 10% of children with mental retardation, 10% of those with cerebral palsy, as well as in large proportions of children with head injuries and with various underlying genetic disorders). There are many forms of epilepsy, each with its own risks to cognitive functioning, and when measuring academic functioning, it is difficult to differentiate the effects of a seizure disorder from the effects of medications used to manage it [20]. Anyway, studies have described higher occurrence of ADHD in children with epilepsy and the reasons for this are not altogether clear but attention difficulties are considered very prevalent in childhood epilepsy. Whatever the cause is, there appears to be a consensus that children with epilepsy are at increased risk for symptoms of inattention [24]. Individuals with both epilepsy and intellectual disability may be at higher risk for significant ADHD symptoms although screening and assessment in children with intellectual disability and epilepsy may be challenging [23]. If there are significant ADHD symptoms associated with childhood epilepsy it is important to determine what real world consequences may result in order to identify possible interventions and provide a rationale for treatment. Hermann et al. (2007) reported that more children with epilepsy and ADHD (69.6%) were provided with other supportive education services compared with children with epilepsy without ADHD (38.5%) [25]. Sherman et al. (2010) reported that children with ADHD and epilepsy had a lower quality of life than children with epilepsy without ADHD. It is clear that both ADHD and epilepsy in childhood are associated with a range of behavioral and affective disorders [26]. It is not clear if the occurrence of both conditions is additive, leading to an even higher risk for psychopathology, although Williams et al. (2003) noted that presence of ADHD in children with epilepsy increased the risk for significant symptoms of anxiety [27]. It seems that children with epilepsy and ADHD are likely to be at higher risk for more negative outcomes in school and in terms of quality of life compared with children with epilepsy alone. Published studies on the treatment of ADHD in childhood epilepsy have focused exclusively on the use of psychopharmacology and particularly methylphenidate (MPH). Although MPH appears to be effective for some children with epilepsy the issue of whether it may lower seizure threshold continues to be debated [23]. In a review of studies of the use of MPH in children with epilepsy it was concluded that the efficacy of MPH in improving symptoms of ADHD was similar to reported rates in children with ADHD without epilepsy and MPH does not adversely affect the severity or frequency of seizures in the individuals with epilepsy, provided they are well controlled for epilepsy [28]. There is a need for more studies focusing on safe and efficacious interventions for symptoms of ADHD in this population [23].

HEADACHE

The prevalence of ADHD among children with chronic headache as well as its association with headache duration and frequency is still contradictory. The two disorders may influence each other simultaneously. Attention difficulties, hyperactivity, inappropriate behavioral symptoms, as well as stress among the family or at school are psychological predictors of headaches. On the other hand, frequent headaches may increase distractibility and further impair learning and attention performance [29]. Literature data suggest that pediatric migraine is associated with impaired attention span and hyperactivity–impulsivity, but not with fully developed ADHD. However, it is interesting to observe that both ADHD and migraine have well-established comorbid connections with epilepsy as well as with mood and anxiety disorders. This has been shown both in clinical and epidemiological studies [30, 31]. There is also evidence for the involvement of dopaminergic systems in the pathophysiology of both disorders, which is one of the possible attractive pathophysiological ways to explain linkage between headaches and ADHD. Other possible explanations have focused on dysfunctional brain iron metabolism, possible genetic linkage, and an underlining common sleep disturbance [32]. Several studies tried to identify alterations of neuronal circuits and cerebral regions which could explain the comorbidity between migraine and ADHD and clarify the association between the two conditions and between them and the different diseases often associated with them, but none provided clear evidence [29]. Today we assume that structural and functional abnormalities in brain networks are central in both chronic headache and ADHD pathophysiology. Therefore, it is important to gain a better understanding of how subcortical–cortical and cortical–cortical network development is altered during the onset and course of these disorders. As in other aspects, treatment modalities in both disorders proved complex and sometimes controversial. On one hand, the first-line drugs used for the treatment of ADHD are stimulants which are generally safe but are associated with adverse effects including headache [33]. On the other hand, cognitive and mental comorbidities affecting patients with chronic headache can increase headache frequency and intensity and therefore should be identified monitored and addressed [34].

ALLERGIC/ATOPIC CONDITIONS AND ASTHMA

Atopic diseases (AD) are common chronic conditions encountered in pediatric clinics. They usually manifest as recurring, noninfectious, inflammatory conditions, and cause a large economic burden despite the development of prevention therapies and medications. As in cognitive processes, it is evident that the development and prevalence of allergic diseases depend on complex interactions between genetic and environmental factors [35]. The etiologies of both AD and ADHD are multifactorial and heterogeneous, which contributes to their development. The increase in prevalence of ADHD diagnoses during the past decades was paralleled by a worldwide increase in atopic and allergic related diseases, such as impetigo. Environmental risk factors that provoke allergic reactions, such as certain food allergens, have been implicated in increasing symptoms of both ADHD and allergic and atopic diseases [36]. A large nationwide, population-based, case-control database from Taiwan display strong and independent associations between ADHD and atopic diseases [35]. The correlations were independent from various factors that are known to have impact on the presence of ADHD.

A possible connection between AD and ADHD is the immune-pathologic hypothesis suggesting that inflammatory cytokines provoked by allergic reactions activate neuro-immune mechanisms, leading to neurobehavioral disorders, including ADHD [37]. Eventually, ADHD was hypothesized as side effects of allergic reactions engendering cholinergic/adrenergic activity imbalance in the neurologic system. Neuro-immunology research suggests dopamine transporters, abundantly expressed on human T cells, are causally implicated in ADHD and are targets for drug like methylphenidate [38]. As a conclusion, ADHD is hypothesized to be an allergic disorder based on a comparison of mechanisms, and hypersensitivity to allergens contributes to the development of ADHD [35].

Another hypothesis regarding the etiologies is that AD and ADHD share common comorbidities, such as sleep disturbance. Studies have explored allergic rhinitis as a risk factor for ADHD. It is known to frequently cause sleep disturbance in childhood and to result in poor concentration and distractive behavior. ADHD causes psychological distress and may be a subsequent, exacerbating factor for atopic conditions, although this conclusion is controversial. Children with ADHD had positive skin prick test results to common allergens consistent with allergic rhinitis. Children with atopic dermatitis have significant sleep problems, which lowers their quality of life [35, 39]. The pathophysiology was proposed as allergic rhinitis subsequent to sinusitis caused by streptococcal infections and caused various pediatric autoimmune neuropsychiatric disorders, including ADHD [40]. Since both disorders are likely to present from early childhood, and possibly be related to immunity through increased exposure to respiratory infections and subsequent neurobehavioral disorders, it seems that signs and symptoms of chronic AD might mask ADHD symptomatology. Since both AD and ADHD Tsai et al. (2013) have mentioned that with regard to the distribution of duration between AD and ADHD, it mostly took 20 to 80 months to diagnose ADHD, which explains why the level of diagnosis of ADHD was lower among preschoolers [35].

The causal results suggest that there are benefits from medication in management of ADHD. Although stimulant drugs are effective for ADHD, managing the associated atopic condition may facilitate improvement of symptoms and minimize medication for children with ADHD [37]. Therefore, the symptoms associated with AD and their medication could play major roles in the management of ADHD symptoms. AD and ADHD could be linked through the histamine pathway, suggesting that antihistamines may be effective for treating ADHD [35, 36]. The potential therapeutic role for antihistamines in ADHD may offer a future alternative treatment choice for patients with dual diagnoses.

Asthma – A study of 102, 253 children from the National Survey of Children's Health showed a twofold increased prevalence of ADHD among children with asthma and even higher rates of ADHD among children with severe asthma [41]. The nature of the relationship between allergic conditions such as asthma and ADHD is not entirely clear. Possible mechanisms underlying this association remain to be investigated but few explanations were given. First, the association could be because of shared risk factors. Low birth weight, impaired fetal growth, and low socioeconomic status are known risk factors for both asthma and ADHD. Second medications used in allergic conditions, such as inhaled corticosteroids were reported as causing altered behavior, hyperactivity and even psychosis in small children, although large studies suggest no evidence of major adverse neuropsychiatric effects. Third, shared strong genetic factors could account for the observed association between allergic conditions ADHD. Mogensen and colleagues (2011) found that 68% of the phenotypic correlation between asthma and hyperactivity-impulsivity was due to genetic influences; thus, a strong genetic component may explain the associations [42]. On the other hand, the results of a study of atopic risk factors for ADHD in the UK General Practice Research Database (GPRD) covering more than 7 million patients support the hypothesis that exposure to foods and inhalants and subsequent type I, immediate (IgE-mediated), hypersensitive mechanisms could play an important role in the causation of ADHD [36]. In this study it was found that there is an increased risk of ADHD in boys with a history of asthma or impetigo and an even stronger risk associated with cow's milk intolerance. These associations were not materially modified by age at first diagnosis. Asthma and impetigo were both common exposures in children with ADHD, whereas cow's milk intolerance was not. Prescription drugs to treat these conditions were also associated with increased risks of ADHD. Histaminergic systems have been implicated in atopic diseases, and pro-inflammatory mechanisms have also been implicated in the development of ADHD. Findings from Pelsser et al. (2009) further support the hypothesis that ADHD may be a hypersensitivity disorder similar to allergy in some children and that allergic and non-allergic forms of ADHD may be distinguished. Such observations might have clinical management implications. There are other options but possible shared etiologic pathways are still not well understood [36, 37]. Whatever the pathophysiologic explanation may be, it seems that in order to reduce the effects of asthma on cognitive performance and ADHD, a multifaceted approach to asthma control and prevention in which primary care providers in the community can and must play a central role, is essential. Coordinated health programs can exert a dramatic influence on asthma morbidity and its cognitive consequences [43].

CELIAC

Celiac disease (CD) is a multisystem disorder triggered by gluten in genetically susceptible individuals. The prevalence in European countries is reported between 1/99–133 [44]. During the past decades, the clinical concept for celiac disease has been expanded, and it is considered a multisystem autoimmune disorder, with most of the patients being asymptomatic, oligosymptomatic, or present with extraintestinal manifestations [45]. In recent years, it has been clear that CD presenting with non-classical signs is more frequent than the classical form. Among the extra-intestinal manifestations, there is a growing body of publications that report neurologic conditions associated with CD, even in asymptomatic patients [46]. Neurologic system complications, perception disorders, and ADHD have been reported in 6% to 11% of patients with CD [47].

There are varied studies about the epidemiology of ADHD among CD patients but confusing data are seen in the literature. While Gongur et al. (2013) reported rates of seropositivity of CD as 1.1% and biopsy-proven CD as 0.27% in a quite large series of children with ADHD. Those figures were not higher than those of normal population. In this study lack of mucosal injury in the majority of seropositive patients and the low degree of damage in patients with ADHD suggest that CD is not be a major concern in children with ADHD [48]. Thus, Gongur et al. (20130) concluded that neither routine screening of CD nor implementation of gluten-free diet in ADHD seems necessary [48]. However, Zelnik et al. (2004) suggested that the variability of neurologic disorders that occur in CD is broader than previously reported and includes "softer" and more common neurologic disorders, such as chronic headache, developmental delay, hypotonia, and ADHD [46]. Niederhofer and Pittschieler (2006) found that that ADHD-like symptomatology is markedly overrepresented among untreated CD outpatients, and that gluten-free diet improves these symptoms significantly. Moreover they have screened the literature and reported a close association of CD, and ADHD symptoms [49].

Most researchers suggest that ADHD-like symptomatology should be included in the list of symptoms of CD [46, 49]. The pathophysiology of the neurological disorders developing in the course of CD is not clear so the issue of response to gluten-free diet is also controversial in patients with neurological disorders [48, 49]. It is agreed that further studies are needed to assess the effect of gluten-free diet and immunomodulation on neurological disorders and to investigate the underlying mechanisms of nervous system involvement associated with gluten sensitivity.

CHRONIC KIDNEY DISEASE

Children with chronic kidney disease (CKD) are at risk for cognitive dysfunction. The etiology of neurocognitive dysfunction in children with CKD is likely multifactorial and may include effects of the renal disease itself as well as effects of associated comorbidities such as anemia, hyperlipidemia, and hypertension. Although advances such as improved nutrition, avoidance of aluminum, improved dialysis, and improved anemia control have significantly decreased the prevalence of severe developmental delay, studies continue to show that children with CKD demonstrate deficits on neurocognitive testing as well as academic achievement that is significantly below grade level in comparison with healthy children [50].

Over half of children with CKD are hypertensive. Given the emerging evidence of neurocognitive deficits in children with primary hypertension, it is plausible that a similar hypertension-cognition link is present in children with hypertension secondary to CKD [51]. Similar effects are seen in studies among children with end-stage kidney disease (ESRD) or severe CKD as well as among children and adolescents with mild-to moderate CKD [51-53]. Kidney transplant is the treatment of choice for children and adolescents with ESRD. It offers life to otherwise fatally ill patients but the trade-off is a lifetime of immunosuppressive drugs, clinic visits and intrusive tests such as biopsies. Immunosuppression carries its own risks by causing susceptibility to infection and malignancies, or sometimes severe side effects [54]. Berney-Martinet et al. (2009) reveals a significantly higher prevalence of psychiatric morbidity (including ADHD), educational impairment and social isolation among adolescents with renal transplant compared to normal controls [54].

Available literature does indicate that children across all stages and all ages of the illness may be vulnerable to cognitive dysfunction, with the degree of dysfunction appearing to correlate with the severity of the illness and not necessarily with age. However, at present, evidence regarding children with mild CKD is limited [53]. However, at present, evidence regarding children with mild CKD is limited. The above described interactions between CKD and different neuro-cognitive aspects including attention are seen among young children as well as adolescents [53, 54].

More specifically, children with CKD have shown relatively lower intellectual capabilities. More specific neuropsychological abilities, such as attention, memory, and selected executive functions, have been shown to be lower when compared with typically developing children who do not have kidney damage [53]. How and why these findings relate to the specific neurocognitive dysfunctions will require additional examination. Although CKD population is a large sample, and although quality of life issues certainly are suspected and have been studied, little data are available documenting the neuro-cognitive concerns. Further, the relatively few studies that exist examining the overall social-behavioral functioning of this population of children indicate little in the way of severe neuro-cognitive disorders. It may be that increased neuro-cognitive difficulties may be present as the illness progresses and/or with the presence of more impaired kidney functions.

CANCER

During the last decades, studies have consistently identified a pattern of neurocognitive deficits, especially attention/concentration difficulties and deficits in executive functioning, in many childhood cancer survivors. Deficits in attention are a significant consequence of the diagnosis and treatment of childhood cancer that affects the central nervous system such as brain tumors and acute lymphoblastic leukemia (ALL) [55]. Most studies have shown that these difficulties may significantly impact the academic performance, social/interpersonal relationships, and vocational success if left unidentified or untreated. As such, it is imperative that researchers focus on understanding the specific nature of these deficits, their precise etiology, and efficacious treatment approaches [56]. To better understand the nature of these deficits, a number of research teams have used an attention-deficit/hyperactivity disorder (ADHD) conceptual framework to guide their research efforts. Findings suggest that indeed many childhood survivors of leukemia and brain tumors evidence attentional difficulties. While risk factors (diagnosis, treatment intensity, time since treatment) may be associated with increased severity of attention deficits, it was concluded that the majority of survivors of pediatric brain tumors and ALL will evidence some degree of impairment affecting daily functioning and quality of life [55, 57].

Among brain tumor survivors, studies have demonstrated that children treated with surgery and standard radiation therapy have developed intellectual decline which is progressive over at least a decade. Risk factors for this cognitive deterioration have been identified and include perioperative complications, possibly hydrocephalus, high radiation dose, large volume radiation, chemotherapy (especially methotrexate), radiation vasculopathy and young age at the time of treatment. In an effort to reduce long-term neurotoxicity, efforts have been made to develop treatment regimens that reduce the impact of these risk factors. Some of these include reduced neuraxis radiation with and without adjuvant chemotherapy, conformal radiation, chemotherapy only protocols for children with optic pathway-hypothalamic tumors and a series of baby brain tumor studies in which chemotherapy (standard and high dose) has allowed radiation to be delayed, reduced or omitted. Whether these changes in therapy will ultimately improve the quality of life of the long-term survivors is uncertain. It is clear that close follow-up of these children is required throughout their lives [57].

Attention problems impact on information processing and encoding, ultimately leading to academic under-performance. Having been successfully used to manage ADHD, stimulants such as methylphenidate (MPH) have been investigated as a beneficial treatment for survivors of childhood cancer. In order to develop appropriate strategies to manage late neurocognitive effects, the results of such trials should be evaluated to identify those children most likely to benefit from stimulants. In a systematic review by Smithson et al. (2013) it was found that short term outcomes for MPH on objective direct measures of attention and parent/teacher ratings of behavior were favorable among children diagnosed and treated due to brain tumors [58]. Observations of side effects indicate that MPH is generally well tolerated in this population. Heterogeneity of study design and outcome measures precluded meta-analysis, so it was concluded that despite yielding only a small number of trials with limited sample size, studies investigating the use of stimulant medication in survivors of childhood brain tumors have provided promising outcomes. Current evidence indicates males, older age when treated, and higher baseline IQ were predictive of greater responsiveness to MPH [58].

Kahalley et al. (2011) have found that attentional deficits experienced by pediatric cancer survivors do not always appear to resemble the clinical presentation of ADHD. Many survivors with cognitive and behavioral difficulties related to attention were not identified using standard ADHD diagnostic approach. Findings offer needed clarification to guide researchers and clinicians in conceptualizing, assessing, and intervening on attentional late effects the diagnostic criteria for ADHD failed to identify many other survivors suffering from post-treatment behavioral dysfunction. It was concluded that conceptualizing attentional late effects as similar to the clinical presentation of ADHD may not be accurate or useful. A common diagnostic difficulty seen in other chronic illnesses is that many survivors experiencing cognitive and behavioral difficulties based on parent and teacher rating scales are not classified as ADHD. This classification finding could imply that a structured clinical interview assessing standard diagnostic criteria for ADHD lacks sensitivity to capture attentional late effects among cancer survivors [59]. Moreover, studies have provided support for the relationship between attention problems and social functioning in survivors of pediatric cancer. Results highlight the need for continued monitoring of both attention problems and difficulties with social functioning in survivors of CNS-impacting pediatric cancer [55].

CHRONIC/CONGENITAL HEART DISEASE

Congenital heart disease (CHD) is the most common birth defect. As treatment for CHD progresses, many more patients are surviving to school age and adulthood. As more children survive with congenital heart disease, their neurodevelopmental outcomes (including ADHD) are becoming increasingly important. It is widely accepted that children with CHD are more likely to suffer from deficiencies in intellectual functioning, developmental difficulties, and problems with academic performance. Children with CHD are at risk for a variety of cognitive deficits, with some demonstrating difficulties in school similar to those of children with disorders of attention. Increased prevalence rates of ADHD among CHD children are high, ranging from 40% to 50% in some studies [60 -62]. The studies suggest that compared with the general population, ADHD may be more prevalent in children with a wide range of CHD, including but not limited to single-ventricle malformations, d-TGA, and total anomalous pulmonary venous connection. Adverse impacts of chronic or intermittent hypoxia on development, behavior, and academic achievement have been reported in studies in children with CHD. Hansen et al. (2012) found that ADHD symptoms are more prevalent in this population of children. Moreover, they have found a trend in this population, towards a greater prevalence of inattention symptoms in patients with cyanosis or single ventricle physiology [63]. Shillingford et al. (2008) found that in a group of children who had undergone cardiac surgery for complex CHD when symptoms of ADHD were scored on the ADHD rating scale 30% of the parents reported high-risk scores for inattention and 29% reported high-risk scores for hyperactivity. They also found that nearly half were using remedial school services. In this study, the presence of cyanosis or single ventricle physiology did not significantly influence the prevalence of ADHD [60].

There are several possible explanations for these findings. Patients born with CHD are exposed to a variety of physiological stressors that continue to change as they mature. Some possible effects of this on the neurological deficits are the level and duration of hypoxemia to which patients with CHD are subjected. Hypoxemia has been found to injure the prefrontal cortex and striate body of the brain. These highly oxygen-sensitive regions are assumed to be associated with the executive control network of attention. In a study by Hovels-Gurich et al. (2007) children who underwent repair of cyanotic tetralogy of Fallot or acyanotic ventricular septal defects in infancy were compared to healthy control subjects. Their data showed that the cyanotic group demonstrated poor attention skills with respect to executive functioning as compared with the acyanotic ventricular septal defect group and the healthy control subjects

[61]. Therefore, it may be possible that risk factors such as cyanosis and single ventricle physiology should be recognized medically for potential family education and intervention of such symptoms, which may affect long-term academic and social development.

Other risk factors included preoperative factors such as microcephaly and seizures, operative factors such as duration of cardiac arrest and rapid de-warming, postoperative factors such as hypoglycemia and seizures, and persistent hypoxemia [64]. Dependency and inactivity, particularly in children with cyanotic lesions, may also play a role in elevated behavioral and attention problems. Parents reported that their own anxiety levels resulted in overprotection of patients and, consequently, limitations of independent behavior [63].

Treatment of ADHD is essential to optimize the child's functioning and to prevent long-term consequences. Optimal diagnosis and management of ADHD are achieved with multimodal interventions that include pharmacotherapy, and psycho-educational interventions. Regulatory decisions regarding ADHD drug licensing and labeling, along with statements from professional associations, raise questions of practice regarding the evaluation and treatment of patients with ADHD. In 2008 the American Heart Association council on cardiovascular disease in the young CHD committee has published a statement recommended electrocardiograms (ECGs) routinely for children before they start medications to treat ADHD [65]. However, the recommendation to obtain an ECG before starting medications for treating ADHD contradicts the carefully considered and evidence based recommendations of the American Academy of Child and Adolescent Psychiatry and the American Academy of Pediatrics. These organizations have concluded that sudden cardiac death in persons taking medications for ADHD is a very rare event, occurring at rates no higher than those in the general population of children and adolescents. Both of these groups also noted the lack of any evidence that the routine use of ECG screening before beginning medication for ADHD treatment would prevent sudden death. The AHA statement pointed out the importance of detecting silent but clinically important cardiac conditions in children and adolescents, which is a goal that the AAP shares. The recommendations of the AAP and the rationale for these recommendations were published later in 2008 [66]. The most recent professional association statement on this issue was published in the European Community by the European Network for Hyperkinetic Disorders, through its European Attention Deficit Hyperactivity Disorder Guidelines Group [67]. A meeting was organized between ADHD specialists, pediatric cardiovascular specialists, and representatives of the major market authorization holders for ADHD medications. In a consensus statement it was claimed that although sudden death has been identified in multiple young individuals on ADHD medication causing regulatory concern, when analyzed for exposure using currently available data, sudden death does not appear to exceed that of the general population. Moreover, it was concluded that there is no current evidence to suggest an incremental benefit to ECG assessment of the general ADHD patient. Since CHD patients have an increased prevalence of ADHD, they can benefit from ADHD proven therapies, including medication. It was also concluded that the ADHD specialist is the appropriate individual to evaluate benefit and risk and recommend therapy in all patients, although discussion with a heart specialist is reasonable for CHD patients. For ADHD patients with suspected heart disease or risk factor/s for sudden death, assessment by a heart specialist is recommended, as would also be the case for a non-ADHD patient. Similar conclusions were stated by the AHA and the final conclusion of both societies is that the identification of risk factors for sudden death should not automatically exclude the use of ADHD medication [67, 68].

So, on the "bottom line", the potential for ADHD (and other developmental disorders) in patients with CHD, even those who undergo early cardiac surgery should be conveyed to parents. The families should be counseled regarding the increased positive screening rate for ADHD in these children and this information should be included in antenatal discussions with parents who have fetuses with antenatally diagnosed CHD [62]. Clinicians who follow this population should screen them for ADHD and follow the AAP and other relevant societies guidelines which provide a useful framework for both evaluation and treatment. Since ADHD is a lifelong disorder and carries significant morbidity, developmental follow-up for this growing population is needed. ADHD is a modifiable condition and appropriate support and intervention can alter the potential outcomes, therefore children with CHD should be screened for ADHD routinely. The formal guidelines suggest that survivors of early cardiac surgery should be evaluated on a case-by-case basis for their eligibility for stimulant medication use.

SUMMARY

Children with chronic illness have medical and cognitive fragility combined with special and sometimes intensive care needs that are not easily met by existing health care and education models. More children than ever in history survive critical medical conditions and suffer from long term chronic disorders. These medical successes in survivorship have likely also resulted in rising rates of complications and childhood chronic needs. These children and their families experience increases in intensive medical technology use, medical and nursing care, and long term coordination needs. Regardless of underlying diagnoses, all these children share similar functional and resource-use consequences, including intensive hospital- and/or community-based service need, reliance on technology, polypharmacy, and/or home care or congregate care to maintain a basic quality of life, risk of frequent and prolonged hospitalizations, which leads to high health resource utilization, and an elevated need for care coordination [69]. Chronic illness affects the lives of many children and their families. The prevalence of illness and disability differs by geographical and economical context. The changing demographic of childhood illness in economically wealthy countries has prompted a re-analysis of the role of pediatric medicine, as chronic illness becomes more prevalent than acute [3, 70]. Usually though a growing number of studies have demonstrated that long-term brain/cognitive dysfunction is common among children with chronic illness, the mechanisms and specific risk factors remain largely unexplained, and sometimes unproven, and may be multifactorial and hard to diagnose [71]. During the past decade, the vast majority of investigations that have examined brain dysfunction have limited their focus to patients with acute critical illness, but it is likely that patients with chronic disease suffer in a more subtle but not less significant ways.

ADHD is an early onset, clinically heterogeneous, complex neurobiological disorder that has been associated with a broad range of impairments including cognitive, academic, behavioral, emotional and social functioning [12]. ADHD is the most common neurodevelopmental disorder of childhood and is among the most prevalent chronic health conditions affecting school-age children [6, 12] it was hypothesized that since chronic diseases are major influential factor regarding cognitive and behavioral processes, and since

ADHD is frequently associated with comorbidities, than chronic disorders should have an effect on the development and course of ADHD in children.

This chapter has discussed the existing published literature that shows widespread negative outcomes of chronic diseases on ADHD and attention performance. Although these children are at risk of poorer health due to the combination of ADHD and chronic illness, there are relatively few well-characterized clinical initiatives and research efforts devoted to improving their care in these aspects. It seems that more work is needed to develop and provide interventions that directly target ADHD of children with chronic illness.

It is suggested that interventions which target specific attention performance and ADHD symptomatology among children with chronic diseases are likely to achieve better results and even might prevent regression and long term comorbidities among these children [70]. Finally, it seems that appropriate research agenda that uses a uniform definition to accurately describe the population and to evaluate outcomes from the perspectives of the child, the family, and the broader health care system is critically needed. With passing years, models of evaluation and treatment of ADHD among children with chronic illness will be further refined, and in turn will help to find successful treatment modalities for this population in need.

REFERENCES

[1]   Wise PH. The future pediatrician: the challenge of chronic illness. *J. Pediatr.* 2007;151(5 suppl):S6 –S10.

[2]   Berry JG, Bloom S, Foley S, Palfrey JS. Health inequity in children and youth with chronic health conditions. *Pediatrics.* 2010;126(Suppl 3):S111-9.

[3]   Van Cleave J, Leslie LK. Approaching ADHD as a chronic condition: implications for long-term adherence. *Pediatr. Ann.* 2008;37:19-26.

[4]   Pastor PN, Reuben CA. Diagnosed attention deficit hyperactivity disorder and learning disability: United States, 2004-2006. *Vital Health Stat.* 2008;237:1-14.

[5]   Wolraich M, Brown L, Brown RT, DuPaul G, Earls M, Feldman HM, Ganiats TG, Kaplanek B, Meyer B, Perrin J, Pierce K, Reiff M, Stein MT, Visser S. Subcommittee on Attention-Deficit/Hyperactivity Disorder; Steering Committee on Quality Improvement and Management, ADHD: clinical practice guideline for the diagnosis, evaluation, and treatment of attention-deficit/hyperactivity disorder in children and adolescents. *Pediatrics.* 2011;128:1007-22.

[6]   Feldman HM, Reiff MI. Clinical practice. Attention deficit-hyperactivity disorder in children and adolescents. *N. Engl. J. Med.* 2014;370:838-46.

[7]   Chan E, Zhan C, Homer CJ. Health care use and costs for children with attention-deficit/hyperactivity disorder: National estimates from the Medical Expenditure Panel Survey. *Arch. Ped. Adolesc. Med.* 2002;156:504-11.

[8]   Coker TR, Elliott MN, Kataoka S, et al. Racial/ethnic disparities in the mental health care utilization of fifth grade children. *Acad. Pediatr.* 2009;9:89-96.

[9]   Betancourt JR, Cervantes MC. Crosscultural medical education in the United States: key principles and experiences. *Kaohsiung J. Med. Sci.* 2009;25:471-8.

[10] Robinson S, Goddard L, Dritschel B, Wisley M, Howlin P. Executive functions in children with Autism Spectrum Disorders. *Brain and Cognition*. 2009;71:362-8.

[11] Hosenbocus S, Chahal R. A review of executive function deficits and pharmacological management in children and adolescents. *J. Can Acad. Child Adolesc. Psychiatry*. 2012;21:223-9.

[12] American Psychiatric Association. Diagnostic and statistical manual of mental disorders: DSM-5. American Psychiatric Association, Washington DC; 2013.

[13] Warikoo N, Faraone SV. Background, clinical features and treatment of attention deficit hyperactivity disorder in children. *Expert Opin. Pharmacother*. 2013;14:1885-906.

[14] Barkley R. 2012. The important role of executive functioning and self-regulation in ADHD. (PDF Document). Retrieved on April 02, 2012, from Russell A. Barkley, Ph.D.: The Official Site: http://www. russellbarkley.org/content/ADHD_EF_ and_SR.pdf.

[15] Rutledge KJ, van den Bos W, McClure SM, Schweitzer JB. Training cognition in ADHD: current findings, borrowed concepts, and future directions. *Neurotherapeutics*. 2012;9:542-58.

[16] Arnsten AF, Rubia K. Neurobiological circuits regulating attention, cognitive control, motivation, and emotion: disruptions in neurodevelopmental psychiatric disorders. *J. Am. Acad. Child Adolesc. Psychiatry*. 2012;51:356-67.

[17] Shaw P, Eckstrand K, Sharp W, et al. Attention-deficit/hyperactivity disorder is characterized by a delay in cortical maturation. *Proc. Natl. Acad. Sci. USA*. 2007;104:19649-54.

[18] Sonuga-Barke EJ, Koerting J, Smith E, et al. Early detection and intervention for attention-deficit/hyperactivity disorder. *Expert Rev. Neurother*. 2011;11:557–63.

[19] Berger I, Nevo Y. Early developmental cues for diagnosis of attention deficit/hyperactivity disorder in young children. *Dev. Disabil Res. Rev*. 2011;17:170-9.

[20] Taras H, Potts-Datema W. Chronic health conditions and student performance at school. *J. Sch. Health*. 2005;75:255-66.

[21] Desrocher M, Rovet J. Neurocognitive correlates of type 1 diabetes mellitus in childhood. *Child Neuropsychol*. 2004;10:36-52.

[22] Chen HJ, Lee YJ, Yeh GC, Lin HC. Association of attention-deficit/hyperactivity disorder with diabetes: a population-based study. *Pediatr Res*. 2013;73:492-6.

[23] Reilly CJ. Attention deficit hyperactivity disorder (ADHD) in childhood epilepsy. *Res Dev Disabil*. 2011;32:883-93.

[24] Dunn DW, Kronenberger WG. Childhood epilepsy, attention problems, and DHD: Review and practical considerations. *Seminars in Pediatric Neurology*. 2006;12:222–8.

[25] Hermann B, Jones J, Dabbs K, Allen CA, Sheth R, Fine J, et al. The frequency, complications and aetiology of ADHD in new onset paediatric epilepsy. *Brain*. 2007;130:3135–48.

[26] Sherman EMS, Brooks BL, Akdag S, Connolly MB, Wiebe S. Parents eport more ADHD symptoms than do teachers in children with epilepsy. *Epilepsy & Behaviour*. 2010;19:428–35.

[27] Williams J, Steel C, Sharp GB, DelosReyes E, Philips T, Bates S, et al. Anxiety in children with epilepsy. *Epilpesy & Behavior*. 2003;4:729–32.

[28] Kaufmann R, Goldberg-Stern H, Shuper A. Attention-deficit disorders and epilepsy in childhood: Incidence, causative relations, and treatment possibilities. *J. Child Neurol.* 2009;24:727–33.

[29] Parisi P, Verrotti A, Paolino MC, Ferretti A, Raucci U, Moavero R, Villa MP, Curatolo P. Headache and attention deficit and hyperactivity disorder in children: Common condition with complex relation and disabling consequences. *Epilepsy Behav.* 2014;32C:72-5.

[30] Jette N, Patten S,Williams J, BeckerW,Wiebe S. Comorbidity ofmigraine and psychiatric disorders — a national population-based study. *Headache.* 2008;48:501–16.

[31] Strine TW, Okoro CA, McGuire LC, Balluz LS. The associations among childhood headaches, emotional and behavioral difficulties, and health care use. *Pediatrics.* 2006;117:1728–35.

[32] Emilien G, Maloteaux JM, Geurts M, Hoogenberg K, Cragg S. Dopamine receptors — physiological understanding to therapeutic intervention potential. *Pharmacol. Ther.* 1999;84:133–56.

[33] Reddy DS. Current pharmacotherapy of attention deficit hyperactivity disorder. *Drugs Today* (Barc). 2013;49:647-65.

[34] Bigal ME, Lipton RB. What predicts the change from episodic to chronic migraine? *Curr. Opin. Neurol.* 2009;22:269-76.

[35] Tsai JD, Chang SN, Mou CH, Sung FC, Lue KH. Association between atopic diseases and attention-deficit/hyperactivity disorder in childhood: a population-based case-control study. *Ann. Epidemiol.* 2013;23:185-8.

[36] Hak E, de Vries TW, Hoekstra PJ, Jick SS. Association of childhood attention-deficit/hyperactivity disorder with atopic diseases and skin infections? A matched case-control study using the General Practice Research Database. *Ann. Allergy Asthma Immunol.* 2013;111:102-6.

[37] Pelsser LM, Buitelaar J, Savelkoul HF. ADHD as a (non) allergic hypersensitivity disorder: a hypothesis. *Pediatr Allergy Immunol.* 2009;20:107-12.

[38] Marshall P. Attention deficit disorder and allergy: a neurochemical model of the relation between the illnesses. *Psychol. Bull.* 1989;106:434-46.

[39] Polanczyk G, de Lima MS, Horta BL, Biederman J, Rohde LA. The worldwide prevalence of ADHD: a systematic review and metaregression analysis. *Am. J. Psychiatr.* 2007;164:942-8.

[40] Chou PH, Lin CC, Lin CH, Loh el-W, Chan CH, Lan TH. Prevalence of allergic rhinitis in patients with attention-deficit/hyperactivity disorder: a population-based study. *Eur. Child Adolesc Psychiatry.* 2013;22:301-7.

[41] Blackman JA, Gurka MJ. Developmental and behavioral comorbidities of asthma in children. *J. Dev. Behav. Pediatr.* 02007;28:92-9.

[42] Mogensen N, Larsson H, Lundholm C, Almqvist C. Association between childhood asthma and ADHD symptoms in adolescence--a prospective population-based twin study. *Allergy.* 2011;66:1224-30.

[43] Basch CE. Asthma and the achievement gap among urban minority youth. *J. Sch. Health.* 2011;81:606-13.

[44] Maki M, Mustalahti K, Kokkonen J, et al. Prevalence of celiac disease among children in Finland. *N. Engl. J. Med.* 2003;348:2517–24.

[45] Branski D, Ashkenazi A, Freier S, et al. Extraintestinal manifestations and associated disorders of celiac disease. *Front Gastrointest Res*. 1992;19:110-21.

[46] Zelnik N, Pacht A, Obeid R, Lerner A. Range of neurologic disorders in patients with celiac disease. *Pediatrics*. 2004;113:1672-6.

[47] Green PH, Alaedini A, Sander HW, et al. Mechanisms underlying celiac disease and its neurologic manifestations. *Cell Mol. Life Sci*. 2005;62:791–9.

[48] Güngör S, Celiloğlu OS, Ozcan OO, Raif SG, Selimoğlu MA. Frequency of celiac disease in attention-deficit/hyperactivity disorder. *J. Pediatr. Gastroenterol. Nutr*. 2013;56:211-4.

[49] Niederhofer H, Pittschieler K. A preliminary investigation of ADHD symptoms in persons with celiac disease. *J. Atten. Disord*. 2006;10:200-4.

[50] Gipson DS, Hooper SR, Duquette PJ, Wetherington CE, Stellwagen KK, Jenkins TL, Ferris ME: Memory and executive functions in pediatric chronic kidney disease. *Child Neuropsychol*. 2006;12:391–405.

[51] Lande MB, Gerson AC, Hooper SR, Cox C, Matheson M, Mendley SR, Gipson DS, Wong C, Warady BA, Furth SL, Flynn JT. Casual blood pressure and neurocognitive function in children with chronic kidney disease: a report of the children with chronic kidney disease cohort study. *Clin. J. Am. Soc. Nephrol*. 2011;6:1831-7.

[52] Hooper SR, Gerson AC, Butler RW, Gipson DS, Mendley SR, Lande MB, Shinnar S, Wentz A, Matheson M, Cox C, Furth SL, Warady BA. Neurocognitive functioning of children and adolescents with mild-to-moderate chronic kidney disease. *Clin. J. Am. Soc. Nephrol*. 2011;6:1824-30.

[53] Gerson AC, Butler R, Moxey-Mims M, Wentz A, Shinnar S, Lande MB, Mendley SR, Warady BA, Furth SL, Hooper SR. Neurocognitive outcomes in children with chronic kidney disease: Current findings and contemporary endeavors. *Ment Retard Dev. Disabil. Res. Rev*. 2006;12:208-15.

[54] Berney-Martinet S, Key F, Bell L, Lépine S, Clermont MJ, Fombonne E. Psychological profile of adolescents with a kidney transplant. *Pediatr Transplant*. 2009;13:701-10.

[55] Moyer KH, Willard VW, Gross AM, Netson KL, Ashford JM, Kahalley LS, Wu S, Xiong X, Conklin HM. The impact of attention on social functioning in survivors of pediatric acute lymphoblastic leukemia and brain tumors. *Pediatr Blood Cancer*. 2012;59:1290-5.

[56] Alderson RM, Mullins LL. Theoretical and clinical implications of using an ADHD framework to understand attention, concentration, and executive functioning deficits in pediatric cancer survivors. *Pediatr Blood Cancer*. 2011;57:4-5.

[57] Duffner PK. Risk factors for cognitive decline in children treated for brain tumors. *Eur. J. Paediatr Neurol*. 2010;14:106-15.

[58] Smithson EF, Phillips R, Harvey DW, Morrall MC. The use of stimulant medication to improve neurocognitive and learning outcomes in children diagnosed with brain tumours: a systematic review. *Eur. J. Cancer*. 2013;49:3029-40.

[59] Kahalley LS, Conklin HM, Tyc VL, Wilson SJ, Hinds PS, Wu S, Xiong X, Hudson MM. ADHD and secondary ADHD criteria fail to identify many at-risk survivors of pediatric ALL and brain tumor. *Pediatr Blood Cancer*. 2011;57:110-8.

[60] Shillingford AJ, Glanzman MM, Ittenbach RF, Clancy RR, Gaynor JW, Wernovsky G. Inattention, hyperactivity, and school performance in a population of school-age children with complex congenital heart disease. *Pediatrics*. 2008;121:e759-67.

[61] Hövels-Gürich HH, Konrad K, Skorzenski D, Herpertz-Dahlmann B, Messmer BJ, Seghaye MC Attentional dysfunction in children after corrective cardiac surgery in infancy. *Ann. Thorac. Surg.* 2007;83:1425-30.

[62] Yamada DC, Porter AA, Conway JL, LeBlanc JC, Shea SE, Hancock-Friesen CL, Warren AE. Early repair of congenital heart disease associated with increased rate of attention deficit hyperactivity disorder symptoms. *Can. J. Cardiol.* 2013;29:1623-8.

[63] Hansen E, Poole TA, Nguyen V, Lerner M, Wigal T, Shannon K, Wigal SB, Batra AS. Prevalence of ADHD symptoms in patients with congenital heart disease. *Pediatr Int.* 2012;54:838-43.

[64] Padula M, Ades A. Neurodevelopmental implications of heart disease. *NeoReviews.* 2006;**7**:e363–9.

[65] Vetter VL, Elia J, Erickson C, et al. Cardiovascular monitoring of children and adolescents with heart disease receiving stimulant drugs: a scientific statement from the American Heart Association Council on Cardiovascular Disease in the Young Congenital Cardiac Defects Committee and the Council on Cardiovascular Nursing. *Circulation.* 2008;117:2407–23.

[66] Perrin JM, Friedman RA, Knilans TK; Black Box Working Group; Section on Cardiology and Cardiac Surgery. Cardiovascular monitoring and stimulant drugs for attention-deficit/hyperactivity disorder. *Pediatrics.* 2008;122:451-3.

[67] Hamilton RM, Rosenthal E, Hulpke-Wette M, Graham JG, Sergeant J; European Network of Hyperkinetic Disorders. Cardiovascular considerations of attention deficit hyperactivity disorder medications: a report of the European Network on Hyperactivity Disorders work group, European Attention Deficit Hyperactivity Disorder Guidelines Group on attention deficit hyperactivity disorder drug safety meeting. *Cardiol. Young.* 2012;22:63-70.

[68] Marino BS, Lipkin PH, Newburger JW, et al. Neurodevelopmental outcomes in children with congenital heart disease: evaluation and management: a scientific statement from the American Heart Association. *Circulation.* 2012;126:1143-72.

[69] Cohen E, Kuo DZ, Agrawal R, Berry JG, Bhagat SK, Simon TD, Srivastava R. Children with medical complexity: an emerging population for clinical and research initiatives. *Pediatrics.* 2011;127:529-38.

[70] Eccleston C, Palermo TM, Fisher E, Law E. Psychological interventions for parents of children and adolescents with chronic illness. *Cochrane Database Syst. Rev.* 2012 Aug 15;8:CD009660.

[71] Girard TD. Brain dysfunction in patients with chronic critical illness. *Respir. Care.* 2012;57:947-5.

In: ADHD

Editors: Itai Berger and Adina Maeir

ISBN: 978-1-63321-047-9

© 2014 Nova Science Publishers, Inc.

Chapter 10

ATTENTION-DEFICIT/HYPERACTIVITY DISORDER AND SUBSTANCE USE DISORDERS

Geurt van de Glind, Ph.D.*

Trimbos-instituut and ICASA Foundation,
Utrecht, the Netherlands

ABSTRACT

Attention-deficit/hyperactivity disorder (ADHD) is highly prevalent in children, adolescents and in adults. Substance Use Disorders (SUD) is ranked in the top of the physical and mental disorders causing the Global Burden of Disease. A growing body of knowledge directs towards a linkage between ADHD and SUD.

Attention-Deficit/Hyperactivity Disorder (ADHD) is a multifactorial determined developmental neuropsychiatric disorder, based on a genetic predisposition and neurobiological deregulations. Substance abuse and dependence are defined as maladaptive patterns of substance use leading to clinically significant impairment or distress.

Extensive research has shown that the adult prognosis for many ADHD-children is poor. Poor outcome was reported in educational performance (higher rates of being disciplined at school; drop out from school; leaving school without diploma; decreased level of higher educational levels), frequent comorbid disorders increased probability of development into antisocial behavior and crime, more frequent and more severe motor vehicle accidents, and higher levels of divorce and underemployment. In addition they more often develop patterns of substance abuse and dependence.

Effective and evidence based treatment options for adolescents and adults with both ADHD and SUD are limited. There is a dramatic lack of good quality research in methods for prevention of SUD-development in ADHD children and adolescents. Hence too few of these methods both for treatment and for prevention are available.

---

* Correspondence: Geurt van de Glind, Ph.D. ICASA Foundation, PO Box 725, 3500 AS Utrecht, the Netherlands; E-mail: gglind@trimbos.nl

INTRODUCTION

Substance use disorders (SUD) are highly prevalent in the general population throughout the world [1-3]. Importantly, Attention Deficit/Hyperactivity Disorder (ADHD) is overrepresented in subjects with SUD in the general population [4, 5], and in clinical samples of patients with SUD [6,7]. In this chapter we will discuss the concepts of both ADHD and SUD. In addition elements of the linkage between ADHD and SUD will be presented, from an etiologic and epidemiologic point of view. The literature on treatment of patients with ADHD and SUD will be reviewed, and finally consequenses for clinical practice and for research will be discussed.

ATTENTION DEFICIT/HYPERACTIVITY DISORDER

Attention-Deficit/Hyperactivity Disorder (ADHD) is a multifactorial determined developmental neuropsychiatric disorder, based on a genetic predisposition and neurobiological dysregulations [8]. The history of the concept goes back to the 18th century and is described by Lange et al., [9]. In 1798, the Scottish physician Alexander Chrichton wrote a book with the title "An inquiry into the nature and origin of mental derangement: comprehending a concise system of the physiology and pathology of the human mind and a history of the passions and their effects". In the chapter "On Attention and its Diseases" he made a clear distinction between normal inattentive behavior and abnormal inattentive behavior, with the latter showing a large overlap with our modern concept of ADHD [10]. In the mid-19th century, the German physician Heinrich Hoffmann wrote "Der Struwwelpeter" [11] (reprint of the 1844 original) or Fidgety Phil in the English version of 1846 (and many reprints thereafter). In both the famous drawings and the story, Fidgety Phil explicitly shows ADHD like behavior.

The start of ADHD in modern science in the beginning of the 20th century is ascribed to Sir George Frederic Still (1868–1941) who presented 20 cases of children with a "defect of moral control as a morbid manifestation, without general impairment of intellect and without physical disease" [12 p. 1079]. He noted: "...a quite abnormal incapacity for sustained attention. Both parents and school teachers have specially noted this feature in some of my cases as something unusual" [12 p. 1166]. Thirty years later, Kramer and Pollnow introduced the concept of Hyperkinetic disease of infancy [13], and listed the inability to sit still for a second, run up and down the room [13 p. 7], climb about preferring high furniture [13 p. 10] and are displeased when deterred from acting out their motor impulses [13 p. 7], concluding that the abnormal motor activity is the main symptom in children with hyperkinetic disease [13 p. 7].

In the 1970s, Ross & Ross [14] discussed brain damage in children with abnormal behavior and in 1980 the concept of Minimal Brain Damage was introduced by Kessler [15].

The same symptoms were, however, already described by Laufer et al., [16] who mentioned that the same behavioral problems can also occur in children without any history or possible brain damage. This lead to the concept of Minimal Brain Dysfunction: "The term minimal brain dysfunction refers to children of near average, average or above average general intelligence with certain learning or behavioral disabilities ranging from mild to severe, which are associated with deviations of function of the central nervous system. These deviations may be manifested by various combinations of impairment in perception, conceptualization, language, memory and control of attention, impulse or motor function" [17 p. 9 f]. Clements further distinguished "[impairment in] control of attention, impulse and motor function" [17 p. 10].

With each iteration of the DSM (DSM-II, DSM-III and III-R), the nomenclature changed. DSM-II introduced the concept of Hyperkinetic reaction of childhood [18], followed by Attention deficit disorder: with and without hyperactivity in DSM-III [19], and then Attention Deficit/Hyperactivity Disorder without a separation between inattentive or hyperactive type in DSM-III-R [20]. In DSM-IV [21], three subtypes were introduced: a predominantly inattentive type, a predominantly hyperactive-impulsive type, and a combined type with symptoms of both pathological dimensions [21]. This edition of the DSM also introduced the diagnosis of adult ADHD.

Though the existence of adult ADHD is widely accepted, the construct and diagnostic criteria of adult ADHD are still under debate [22-24]. Some years ago, Barkley et al., [25] highlighted several problems related to both childhood ADHD (focused on boys rather than girls; symptoms overlap with other psychiatric disorders) and adult ADHD (symptoms are related to children rather than to adults) in DSM-IV. According to Barkley et al. [25], these problems resulted in the suggested underdiagnosis of adult ADHD due to the requirement of an equal number of symptoms (6 out of 9) for the symptom criterion for childhood and for adult ADHD [25]. Despite these serious problems, changes in ADHD-criteria for DSM-5 are relatively minor [26] and the wording of the 18 symptoms will not be changed, but for adults there will be examples related to adult behavior embedded in the description of symptoms. However, a rather important change for adult ADHD in DSM-5 is the higher Age of onset criterion: some of the symptoms must be present before age 12 (compared to age 7 in DSM-IV-TR) [27]. In addition, the Number of symptoms criterion for adults has been changed to 5 out of 9 symptoms (compared to 6 out of 9 in DSM-IV-TR) for both of the inattentive and hyperactive/impulsive symptoms [26].

ETIOLOGY

It is beyond the scope of this chapter to extensively describe and discuss the etiology of ADHD. Instead, we will briefly present those etiological factors that may be of relevance for the observed link between ADHD and SUD.

In general, as for all of the psychiatric and developmental disorders, there is no single factor causing ADHD. In the literature several interdependent biological (genetic/neurobiology) and psychosocial/environmental factors can be found [28-30]. Recent neuroimaging studies have shown an altered brain structure and function in specific brain circuits related to the regulation of attention, inhibition/cognitive control, motivation/reward, and emotion [29, 31]. For example, children with ADHD showed prominent abnormalities in the inferior prefrontal cortex and its connections to striatal, cerebellar, and parietal regions [31, 32].

In a recent comprehensive review it is stated that ADHD is familial and highly heritable [30]. However the question by what route or routes (exposure to psychosocial/ environmental factors) the vulnerability for ADHD leads to inattentive and/or hyperactive/impulsive behavior, and ultimately to the disorder, has not yet been answered. Even more, it is concluded that "there is a large literature documenting associations between ADHD and a wide variety of putative environmental risks that can, at present, only be regarded as correlates" [30 p. 3). Finally, a significant association between anhedonia and inattentive symptoms of ADHD has been found, suggesting a reward insensitivity problem in ADHD [33].

LONG TERM OUTCOME OF ADHD

Extensive research has shown that the adult prognosis for many ADHD-children is poor. Poor outcome was reported in educational performance (higher rates of being disciplined at school; drop out from school; leaving school without diploma; decreased level of higher educational levels), frequent comorbid disorders (including SUD), increased probability of development into antisocial behavior and crime, more frequent and more severe motor vehicle accidents, and higher levels of divorce and underemployment [25, 28]. Furthermore, decreased work productivity was reported: 22 more work loss days per year in ADHD subjects compared to non ADHD subjects according to the WHO World Mental Health Survey Initiative, with data from 10 countries [34].

SUBSTANCE USE DISORDERS

Substance abuse and dependence are defined as maladaptive patterns of substance use leading to clinically significant impairment or distress [21]. Van den Brink and Schippers [35] gave an overview of the changing paradigms related to substance abuse and dependence. They more or less chronically listed the Moral Model (moral weakness constitutes the basis of habitual drunkenness and thus addiction is a choice and a person's own responsibility), the Pharmacological Model (the addictive nature of the substance leads to addiction), the Symptomatic Model (substance abuse is not a disorder in itself, but it represents a symptom of an underlying character or personality disorder), the Disease Model (with uncontrolled substance use and tolerance as main concepts, leading to the view that abstinence should be the target for treatment), the Psychological Model (substance abuse is a form of learned maladaptive behavior, hence treatment is based on a remodeling of the behavioral patterns involved), and the Social Model (substance abuse is a normal reaction to abnormal circumstances and treatment should be directed to a change in the environment). In 1976, these different models were integrated in the Bio-Psycho-Social Model proposed by Edwards and Gross [36] using the concept of the substance dependence syndrome [37]. According to this model, addiction is the result of an interaction between genetic/biological vulnerabilities, psychological characteristics and environmental factors. Since the early 1990's, the biological aspects of this model are considered to be of crucial importance, leading to the view that addiction is a disease of the brain [38]. In their landmark paper, McLellan et al., [39] presented convincing evidence that substance dependence is a chronic disease like diabetes, hypertension, and asthma and that substance dependence "should be insured, treated and evaluated like other chronic illnesses" [39 p.1689]. Recently, however, Arria and McLellan [40] noted that this approach has not resulted in sufficient changes in addiction treatment.

To summarize, addiction is currently conceptualized as a chronic relapsing brain disorder with a complex biopsychosocial etiology and the phenotype in current classification systems (DSM-IV; ICD-10) closely resembles the dependence syndrome developed by Edwards and Gross [36]. However, some changes have been made in the classification of addiction in the most recent edition of the DSM: DSM-5 [26].

The three most prominent changes in the description of the phenotype of addiction in DSM-5 are: 1) inclusion of behavioral addictions in the chapter of 'Addiction and Related Disorders'; 2) removal of the 'committing illegal acts' criterion and addition of a 'craving' criterion from the menu of symptoms belonging to the core concept of addiction; and 3) elimination of the abuse/dependence dichotomy and combining the symptoms of these disorders into one disorder with different levels of severity. These changes are generally consistent with the original formulation of the dependence syndrome and are thought to be instrumental in the diagnosis and treatment of substance use and related disorders [41 p. 106].

It is beyond the scope of this chapter to fully discuss the etiology of SUD. Here we only mention those elements of the etiology that are of importance for the link between SUD and ADHD.

Although there is growing knowledge about why some individuals become addicted when exposed to drugs or alcohol, whereas others do not, much is still unknown. The literature shows strong evidence for the role of genetic risks [42], neurobiological vulnerabilities [43,44], and certain developmental and environmental factors [45] influencing the genetic and neurobiological vulnerability for and the development of SUD.

Environmental factors are considered more important for initiation and less important for progression to dependence. The reverse is true for genetic factors [42].

Neurobiological features, such as motivation and reward and impaired ability to inhibit intentional actions, are highly relevant as vulnerability factors for the development of SUD [46]. In addition, some authors also suggests an association between anhedonia or reward deficiency (i.e., diminished pleasure following natural reward) and the development of stimulant dependence [47-50].

The dopamine system is strongly involved in expecting and experiencing pleasure, and in feeling good. Hence it is involved in conditioning via motivation and reward [44]. Impairments in the motivation and reward system and in the ability to inhibit intentional actions have major implications for social functioning, adding to the risk to develop a SUD [44, 46, 51, 52].

In discussing social factors and biological and psychological factors, Glantz and Pickens [53 p. 9] state: "In general, drug use appears to be more a function of social and peer factors, whereas drug abuse appears to be more a function of biological and psychological processes". The complex and individually tailored pattern of risk factors for the development of SUD is also discussed by Sloboda et al., [45]. They emphasize the interaction between vulnerabilities and (groups of) risk factors and conclude that "This interaction is bidirectional, i.e., it promotes social selection (e.g., forming friendships with peers having similar characteristics) and social contagion (e.g., influence of peers on individual behavior)" [45 p. 947].

PREVALENCE

Alcohol Use Disorders

There is a causal relationship between alcohol consumption and the global burden of disease: "The net effect of alcohol consumption on health is detrimental, with an estimated 3•8% of all global deaths and 4•6% of global disability-adjusted life-years attributable to alcohol. Disease burden is closely related to average volume of alcohol consumption, and is strongest in poor people and in those who are marginalized from society. The costs associated with alcohol amounts to more than 1% of the gross national product in high-income and middle-income countries, with the costs of social harm constituting a major proportion in addition to health costs" [1 p. 2223].

In 2005, 45.8% of the adult world population was a lifetime alcohol abstainer, 13.8% had drank before but was currently abstaining from alcohol, and 40.6% was a current drinker. On average, current drinkers consumed 17.1 liters of pure alcohol per year [2]. Shield and colleagues conclude that "lifetime abstention was most prevalent in North Africa, the Middle East and South Asia" and that "the prevalence of abstention, level of alcohol consumption and patterns of drinking vary widely across regions of the world", with Europe having the lowest abstention rates and the highest consumption levels [2 p. 2]. In their study extrapolating German figures and costs on alcohol and nicotine consumption to the European Union, Effertz and Mann [54] conclude that "substance use disorders rank on top of all disorders of the brain in Europe" [54 p. 1]. An alcohol use disorder is present in 14.6 million European citizens, representing 3.4% of the adult population [55].

Drug Use Disorders

Degenhardt and Hall [3] estimated that 149–271 million people used an illicit drug worldwide in 2009 of which 125–203 million (75-85%) were cannabis users; 15–39 million (10-15%) were problem users of opioids, amphetamines, or cocaine, and 11–21 million (10-15%) injected drugs. They state that the levels of illicit drug use seem to be highest in high-income countries and in countries near major drug production areas. However, there are very limited reliable data for illicit drug use in low-income countries.

THE LINKAGE BETWEEN ADHD AND SUD

The following questions will be explored in this paragraph:

1) What is the prevalence of ADHD in SUD populations?
2) What is known about the causes of the relation between ADHD and SUD?
3) What is known about comorbidity patterns in treatment seeking SUD populations with and without ADHD?

1) Prevalence

Recently, Van Emmerik-van Oortmerssen et al., [6] presented the results of a meta-analysis on 12 prevalence studies in adult treatment seeking SUD patients. Eight out of 12 studies were conducted in the USA. A prevalence of ADHD in these individual studies was reported, ranging from 10.0% to 54.1%. The variability in findings was partly explained by the primary substance of abuse and by the difference in diagnostic instrument.

We performed an international multi-center cross sectional study on ADHD in treatment seeking SUD patients, the International ADHD in Substance use disorders Prevalence (IASP) study [56]. In one part of this study [7] we found a range of 4% to 10% of DSM-IV ADHD in outpatient Alcohol Use Disorder subjects and a range of 12% to 30% in outpatient Drug Use Disorder subjects in non-Nordic countries, with slightly higher rates for DSM-5, and substantial higher rates for Nordic countries (Sweden and Norway).

Even in participating centers with the lowest prevalence estimate of adult ADHD (5% in an AUD treatment center in Hungary and Switzerland), the rates were twice the pooled prevalence rate for adult ADHD in the general population: 2.5% [57].

2) Risk for the Development of SUD in ADHD Children

In their review of longitudinal studies of ADHD children followed up into adulthood, Lee et al., [58] summarized the increased risk of SUD in ADHD children compared to non-ADHD controls as follows:

1)   ever having used nicotine (OR=2.08, CI=1.66-2.60, p<.001);
2)   ever having used marijuana (OR=2.78, CI=1.64-4.74, p<.001);
3)   marijuana abuse or dependence (OR=1.58, CI=1.16-2.14, p=.003);
4)   alcohol use disorder (OR=1.74, CI=1.38-2.20, p<.001);
5)   cocaine abuse or dependence in adolescence/adulthood (OR=2.05, CI=1.38-3.04, p<.001); and
6)   overall drug abuse/dependence based on studies without an explicit specification of the primary substance of abuse (OR=2.64, CI=1.77-3.94, p<.001).

Explanatory Models
Pathway via development of Antisocial Personality Disorder
In their review, Flory and Lynam [59] presented four models for the relation between externalizing disorders, SUD and the role of ADHD:

1)   ADHD is not an independent risk factor, and the risk related to ADHD is attenuated or disappears after controlling for the presence of Conduct Disorder (CD). Thus, the development of SUD is accounted for by comorbid Oppositional Defiant Disorder (ODD) and/or Conduct Disorder (CD) [60-62, 5];
2)   ADHD is an important and independent risk factor for the development of SUD, especially for nicotine use and dependence [63-65];

3) ADHD is a risk factor for the development of CD and then SUD development in subjects with CD kicks in [59];

4) The combination of ADHD and CD accounts for more severe patterns of SUD than either one of these disorders alone.; a model that was recently confirmed in heroin dependent patients [66, 67, 59]

It is not known yet which model or which combination of models represents the real world relationship between ADHD and SUD in the most comprehensive way. However, the important, but non-replicated, results reported by Elkins et al. [68] provide at least a good start in our thinking about the relationship between ADHD and SUD. They included 1,404 11 year old general population children (694 boys) and assessed them three times: at baseline (11 years), at 14 years and at 18 years. They looked for categorical diagnoses of ADHD and CD and for dimensional measures of ADHD (inattentive vs. hyperactive/impulsive scores) and CD and tested how these categorical and dimensional measures influenced the presence of SUD at age 18. Interestingly the categorical diagnosis of ADHD at 11 years predicted only nicotine dependence at age 18, but when adjusted for the presence of CD, the significance of this finding disappeared.

However, the dimensional measures of hyperactivity/impulsivity predicted the presence of both nicotine dependence and cannabis abuse and dependence and these effects remained significant after controlling for CD [68]. They also reported significant values for the prediction of SUD for even 1 symptom of ADHD or CD. These findings were supported by results of a recent study in adolescents with ADHD, with hyperactive/impulsive symptoms predicting smoking [69].

Lee and colleagues concluded that the current prospective literature on the link between ADHD and SUD and the role of CD is too scarce to conclude that ADHD does not play an important independent role in the development of SUD [58].

The literature suggests that ADHD is probably an independent risk factor for tobacco dependence and probably Drug Use Disorders (DUD), but this might not be the case for Alcohol Use Disorders (AUD). However, the greatest risk is of the development of SUD is for youngsters with a comborbid diagnosis of CD and ADHD, leading to greater a risk for almost every SUD than the presence of a diagnosis of either CD or ADHD alone [70].

Neurobiological Model of Overlap between ADHD and SUD

Recent studies have shown common genetic vulnerabilities for SUD, ADHD and other externalizing disorders [71]. As presented in some of the previous paragraphs, also similar brain functions and brain-structures are involved in both SUD [43, 44] and ADHD [29, 31, 32], including brain areas involved in inhibition, motivation and reward and more general the dopamine system.

In addition, there are similarities in ADHD and SUD in terms of dysfunctional inhibitory processes. What remains unclear is whether the lack of inhibition among those with ADHD is what increases risk for SUD. What is probably true is that once someone has a SUD, deregulation of the inhibitory system is exacerbated by the excessive use of alcohol and/or drugs [70].

3) Comorbidity Patterns

SUD in treatment seeking subjects is often comorbid with other psychiatric disorders such as Major Depression, Bipolar Disorder, Anxiety Disorders, Borderline, Schizophrenia and Antisocial Personality Disorder [72-75]. Adult ADHD is also associated with high rates of comorbid disorders such as Mood and Anxiety Disorders, and Antisocial Personality Disorders [76-78]. Moreover, for those with both ADHD and SUD there is an even further increased risk for comorbidity with Mood and Anxiety Disorders and for Antisocial Personality Disorders [66, 79-81].

In our IASP study [82] we found that treatment seeking SUD patients with ADHD showed more psychiatric comorbidity than those without ADHD: Antisocial personality disorder, borderline personality disorder, current major depression and current (hypo)manic episode were all significantly more prevalent in SUD patients with ADHD compared to SUD patients without ADHD. In SUD patients with ADHD 75% had at least one additional comorbid disorder compared to "only" 37% of SUD patients without ADHD. This study was the first to look at comorbidity patterns in ADHD subtypes in treatment seeking SUD patients. Comorbidity patterns differed between ADHD subtypes with increased MD in the inattentive and combined ADHD subtype (p<.01), increased HME and APD in the hyperactive/impulsive ADHD subtype (p<.01) and the combined ADHD subtype (p<.001) and increased BPD in all three subtypes (p<.001). These differences were in line with research suggesting underlying pathofysiology for SUD and comorbid disorders [83, 70] and research showing empirical evidence for the distinction between internalizing and externalizing psychiatric and personality disorders [42].

TREATMENT OF PATIENTS WITH ADHD AND SUD

Efficacy of the pharmacological treatment in adult ADHD is well documented and reviewed, concluding that such treatment has robust positive effects on reducing ADHD symptoms [84-86] with better effects for stimulant medication compared to non-stimulant medication [86]. In contrast, data on the non-pharmacological treatment of ADHD in adults is limited but also indicates positive effects of non-pharmacological treatment options [87-89] . The NICE practice guideline on ADHD concludes on treatment of adult ADHD: "Currently there is good evidence supporting the effectiveness of methylphenidate in people with ADHD symptoms and associated impairment. However, there is insufficient evidence on whether non-drug treatments could have specific advantages in some important aspects of the life of a person with ADHD. Given the strong association of ADHD in adults with substance misuse, personality disorder and involvement in the criminal justice system, a health economic approach would be essential" [90 p. 45-46].

However, stimulant treatment of adult ADHD in patients with SUD is much less effective than in adult ADHD patients without SUD in the reduction of ADHD symptoms ant it also has little effect on substance use [91]. In his review, Carpentier [91] looked at all controlled studies in this population and found a small effect for stimulant medication on ADHD symptoms in only one study in adults [92], in only one study in adolescents [93] and small effects on secondary ADHD outcome measures in one study in adolescents [94]. Carpentier

[91] also reported a moderate effect of atomoxetine on ADHD symptoms in one study in adults with alcohol dependence [95]. The same study was also the only one with a small effect on alcohol use. Two studies reported small effect sizes on secondary outcome measures for SUD outcome, one in adults [96] and one in adolescents [94]. Four studies showed no significant result in neither ADHD nor SUD [97-100]. Explanations for these results have been proposed but scarcely tested.

Carpentier [91] points to several possible explanations for these results: 1) the high prevalence of additional comorbidity in populations with ADHD and addiction; 2) diagnostic inaccuracy; 3) effects of long-term psychoactive substances on the brain and on its responsiveness to ADHD medication; 4) inadequate medication dosages; and 5) the "classic pattern of dual disorder treatment" in which "active treatment alleviates the comorbid disorder but does not directly influence the SUD" [91 p. 19]. Crunelle et al., [101] tested whether a low dopamine transporter occupancy by methylphenidate could be a possible reason for reduced treatment effectiveness in ADHD patients with and without cocaine dependence, using single photon emission computed tomography (SPECT). However, they had to reject their hypothesis, suggesting that higher doses of methylphenidate are not very likely to improve the effectiveness of stimulants in patients with ADHD and comorbid SUD.

Recently a study has been performed by Konstenius and colleagues [102] with titration to (when necessary) high dosages of stimulants in imprisoned male patients with ADHD and SUD. She found effects on both ADHD and SUD outcome measures.

To the best of our knowledge, there are no results of non-pharmaceutical treatment options for ADHD in SUD patients available. Recently, van Emmerik-van Oortmerssen and colleagues proposed integrated CBT treatment for this population [103].

In addition to the above mentioned reasons for the small or absent effects in the treatment of ADHD in SUD patients [91, 101], the chosen outcome measures and the duration of trials should be considered.

The current outcome measures (e.g., level of ADHD symptoms; abstinence of substance use; level of substance use at a given moment) in all controlled research so far may not be the most suitable and sensitive in this specific population. Other outcome measures such as criminality [104] and injuries [105] may be of importance. Moreover, so far, with the exception of Konstenius et al., [102] only fixed dosages have been used in previous trials [91]. Individually tailored dosages of ADHD medication are known to be of importance in treatment of adult ADHD [106, 102]. Using titration, but also using responders and non-responders may be considered in developing designs and methods for future trials.

Hence, we should seek for clever and novel research designs and new outcome parameters to test and, if needed, develop effective treatments for subjects suffering from both ADHD and SUD.

PREVENTION OF SUD DEVELOPMENT IN ADHD CHILDREN AND ADOLESCENTS

In an extensive systematic review and meta-analysis, investigating the long-term outcome of ADHD subjects with and without pharmacological treatment, Shaw and colleagues [29] conclude, that those without treatment had poorer outcome (including more SUD), when compared to those who were treated for ADHD, although significant differences remained also for this group when compared to healthy controls [29]. Fredriksen et al., [85] reviewed the literature on the effect of stimulant treatment of ADHD children/ adolescents for the development of SUD. There is a clear protective effect, but this effect seems to decrease over the years, due to so far unknown reasons. Family related factors, other environmental factors, and limited adherence to the medication are all possible explanations [85].

CONSEQUENSES FOR CLINICAL PRACTICE

The phenomenon of ADHD presence in SUD patients can no longer be attributed to a USA hype or to biased USA scientific work. Hence, professionals and managers of addiction treatment centers worldwide should work on the detection, diagnosis and treatment of these patients. The severity and consequences for quality of life of both disorders demand this. In addition, in the field of adolescent addiction treatment, professionals should be aware of possible comorbid ADHD.

Short term and long term collaboration between clinical practice and science is warranted for a further improvement of the quality and effectiveness of existing and new diagnostic and treatment procedures, both in adolescents and adults.

Finally, in the fields of child and adolescent psychiatry and youth care, professionals should be aware of the risk for development of SUD in ADHD children and adolescents. Together with people from the clinical field, scientists should develop and test methods for prevention of SUD in children, adolescents and in (young) adults with ADHD.

CONCLUSION

Many children with ADHD grow up with serious consequences such as educational problems, other psychiatric disorders, social/relationship problems, occupational problems, motor vehicle accidents, suicidal behavior and suicide, and excessive substance use or SUD in later life. Prospective studies of children with ADHD, with a follow up into adulthood, show this increased risk for SUD. However there is debate on the role of comorbid CD and the development of Antisocial Personality Disorder (APD). Some of the researchers therefore conclude that ADHD is not an independent risk factor for the development of SUD and that comorbid CD during adolescence and APD in adulthood fully account for this risk. A growing consensus emerges that ADHD affects the course of SUD in such a way that the latter has a more chronic, complex and severe course in CD+ADHD subjects than in subjects with either CD or ADHD only. A minority of studies conclude that ADHD is an independent risk factor [58, 59]. However, so far only one of the studies differentiated between the causal role of ADHD subtypes, i.e., the different role of inattention and hyperactive/impulsive symptoms. This study found that impulsive/hyperactive symptoms of ADHD were a strong independent risk factor for SUD development [68].

Since we are only beginning to understand the relationship between ADHD and SUD, more research is warranted in many research domains to solve the ADHD-SUD puzzle. This is of crucial importance to find effective methods for prevention of SUD development in ADHD children and adolescents.

There is little evidence for effectiveness of medicinal treatment of ADHD in SUD patients. And there has been hardly any research performed so far on non-medicinal treatment options for this population. Neither for adults, nor for adolescents. This lack of treatment options for clinicians should be filled with evidence based interventions. Hence researchers and clinicians should work on filling this gap.

REFERENCES

[1]   Rehm, J., Mathers, C., Popova, S., Thavorncharoensap, M., Teerawattananon, Y., Patra, J. (2009). Global burden of disease and injury and economic cost attributable to alcohol use and alcohol use disorders. *Lancet*, 373(9682), 2223-2233. doi: 10.1016/S0140-6736(09).

[2]   Shield, K. D., Rylett, M., Gmel, G., Gmel, G., Kehoe-Chan, T.A., Rehm, J. (2013). Global alcohol exposure estimates by country, territory and region for 2005 - a contribution to the Comparative Risk Assessment for the 2010 Global Burden of Disease Study. *Addiction*, 108(5), 912-922. doi:10.1111/add.12112.

[3]   Degenhardt, L., & Hall, W. (2012). Extent of illicit drug use and dependence, and their contribution to the global burden of disease. *Lancet*, 379(9810), 55-70. doi: 10.1016/S0140-6736(11)61138-0.

[4]   Kessler, R. C., Adler, L. A., Barkley, R., Biederman, J., Conners, C. K., Faraone, S. V., Greenhill, L. L., Jaeger, S., Secnik, K., Spencer, T., Ustün, T. B., Zaslavsky, A. M. (2005). Patterns and predictors of attention-deficit/hyperactivity disorder persistence into adulthood: results from the national comorbidity survey replication. *Biological psychiatry, 57*(11), 1442-1451.

[5]   Tuithof, M., ten Have, M., van den Brink, W., Vollebergh, W., de Graaf, R. (2012). The role of conduct disorder in the association between ADHD and alcohol use (disorder). Results from the Netherlands Mental Health Survey and Incidence Study-2. *Drug and Alcohol Dependence*, 123(13), 115-121. doi: 10.1016/j.drugalcdep.2011.10.030.

[6]   Van Emmerik-van Oortmerssen, K., Van de Glind, G., Van den Brink, W., Smit, F., Crunelle, C. L., Swets, M., Schoevers, R. A. (2012). Prevalence of attention-deficit hyperactivity disorder in substance use disorder patients: A meta-analysis and meta-regression analysis. *Drug and Alcohol Dependence*, 122(1-2), 11-19.

[7]   van de Glind, G., Konstenius, M., Koeter, M.W., van Emmerik-van Oortmerssen, K., Carpentier, P.J., Kaye, S., Degenhardt, L., Skutle, A., Franck, J., Bu, E.T., Moggi, F., Dom, G., Verspreet, S., Demetrovics, Z., Kapitány-Fövény, M., Fatséas, M., Auriacombe, M., Schillinger, A., Møller, M., Johnson, B., Faraone, S.V., Ramos-Quiroga, J.A., Casas, M., Allsop, S., Carruthers, S., Schoevers, R.A., Wallhed, S., Barta, C., Alleman, P., Levin, F.R., van den Brink, W.; IASP Research Group. (2014). Variability in the prevalence of adult ADHD in treatment seeking substance use disorder patients: results from an international multi-center study exploring DSM-IV and DSM-5 criteria. *Drug Alcohol Depend*. 2014 Jan 1;134:158-66. doi: 10.1016.

[8]   8. Kieling, R., & Rohde L.A., (2012). ADHD in Children and Adults: Diagnosis and Prognosis. In: Stanford C, & Tannock R, (eds). Behavioral Neuroscience of Attention Deficity Hyperactivity Disorder and Its Treatment. *Current Topis in Behavioral Neurosciences* 9. New York: Springer. pp 1-16.

[9]   Lange, K. W., Reichl, S, Lange, K. M., Tucha, L., Tucha O. (2010).The history of attention deficit hyperactivity disorder. *Attention Deficit Hyperactivity Disorder*, 2(4), 241–255. doi: 10.1007/s12402010-0045-8.

[10]   Crichton, A. (1798). An inquiry into the nature and origin of mental derangement: comprehending a concise system of the physiology and pathology of the human mind and a history of the passions and their effects. *Journal of Attention Disorders*, 12, 200–204.

[11]   Hoffmann, H. (1948). Der Struwwelpeter. Oder lustige Geschichten und drollige Bilder für Kinder von 3 bis 6 Jahren. Loewes, Stuttgart: Frankfurter Originalausgabe.

[12]   Still, G. F. (1902). Some abnormal psychical conditions in children: the Goulstonian lectures. *Lancet*, 1, 1008–1012.

[13]   Kramer, F., & Pollnow, H., (1932). Über eine hyperkinetische Erkrankung im Kindesalter. Aus der Psychiatrischen und Nerven-Klinik der Charité in Berlin (Direktor: Geh. Med.-Rat Prof. Dr. Bonhoeffer) *Mschr Psychiat Neurol*, 82, 21-40. doi: 10.1159/000164074.

[14]   Ross, D. M., & Ross, S. A., (1976). Hyperactivity: research, theory and action. New York: Wiley.

[15]   Kessler, J. W. (1980). History of minimal brain dysfunctions. In: Rie HE, Rie ED, editors. Handbook of minimal brain dysfunctions: a critical view. New York: Wiley; pp. 18–51.

[16]   Laufer, M. W., Denhoff, E., Solomons, G. (1957). Hyperkinetic impulse disorder in children's behavior problems. *Psychosomatic Medicine*, 19, 38–49.

[17]   Clements, S. D. (1966). Minimal brain dysfunction in children: terminology and identification: phase one of a three-phase project. Washington DC: US Department of Health, Education and Welfare.

[18]   American Psychiatric Association. (1968). Diagnostic and statistical manual of mental disorders (DSM-II) 2. Washington DC: American Psychiatric Association.

[19]   American Psychiatric Association. (1980). Diagnostic and statistical manual of mental disorders (DSM-III) 3. Washington DC: American Psychiatric Association.

[20]   American Psychiatric Association. (1987). Diagnostic and statistical manual of mental disorders (DSM-III-R), 3rd edn rev. Washington DC: American Psychiatric Association.

[21]   American Psychiatric Association. (1994). Diagnostic and Statistical Manual of Mental Diseases (DSM-IV). Vol 4th ed. Washington, DC: 1994.

[22]   Fischer, M., & Barkley, R. A. (2007). The persistence of ADHD into adulthood: (once again) it depends on whom you ask. *The ADHD Report*, 15(4) ,7–16. doi: 10.1521/adhd.2007.15.4.7.

[23]   Solanto, M. V., Wasserstein. J., Marks, D.J., Mitchell, K.J.J. (2012). Diagnosis of ADHD in adults: what is the appropriate DSM-5 symptom threshold for hyperactivity-impulsivity? *Attention Disorders*, 16(8), 631-634. doi: 10.1177/1087054711416910.

[24]   Kessler, R. C., Green, J. G., Adler, L. A., Barkley, R. A., Chatterji, S., Faraone, S.V ., Finkelman, M., Greenhill, L. L., Gruber, M. J., Jewell, M., Russo, L. J., Sampson, N.

A., Van Brunt, D. L. (2010). Structure and diagnosis of adult attention-deficit/hyperactivity disorder: analysis of expanded symptom criteria from the Adult ADHD Clinical Diagnostic Scale. *Archives of General Psychiatry*, 67(11), 1168-78. doi: 10.1001/archgenpsychiatry.2010.146.

[25] Barkley R. A., Murphy K. R., & Fischer M. (2008). ADHD in Adults: What the Science Says. New York: The Guilford Press.

[26] American Psychiatric Association. (2013). *Highlights of Changes from DSM-IV-TR to DSM-5. 2013.* http://www.psych.org/practice/dsm/dsm5 [Accessed 21st April 2013].

[27] Dalsgaard, S. (2013). Attention-deficit/hyperactivity disorder (ADHD). European Child & Adolescent Psychiatry, 22(Suppl:1), 43-48. doi: 10.1007/s00787-012-0360-z.

[28] Nigg, J. (2012). Environment, developmental origins, and attention-deficit/hyperactivity disorder. *Archives of Pediatrics and Adolescent Medicine*, 166(4), 387-388.

[29] Shaw, M., Hodgkins, P., Caci, H., Young, S., Kahle, J., Woods, A. G., Arnold, L. E. (2012). A systematic review and analysis of long-term outcomes in attention deficit hyperactivity disorder: effects of treatment and non-treatment. *BMC Medicine*, 10, 99.

[30] Thapar, A., Cooper, M., Eyre, O., Langley, K. (2013). What have we learnt about the causes of ADHD? *Journal of Child Psychology and Psychiatry*, 54(1), 3-16.

[31] Arnsten, A. F., & Rubia, K. (2012). Neurobiological circuits regulating attention, cognitive control, motivation, and emotion: disruptions in neurodevelopmental psychiatric disorders. *Journal of the American Academy of Child & Adolescent Psychiatry*, 51(4), 356-367. doi: 10.1016/j.jaac.2012.01.008.

[32] Cubillo, A., Halari, R., Smith, A., Taylor, E., Rubia, K. (2012). A review of fronto-striatal and fronto cortical brain abnormalities in children and adults with Attention Deficit Hyperactivity Disorder (ADHD) and new evidence for dysfunction in adults with ADHD during motivation and attention. *Cortex*, 48(2), 194–215.

[33] Meinzer, M. C., Pettit, J. W., Leventhal, A. M., Hill, R. M. (2012). Explaining the covariance between attention-deficit hyperactivity disorder symptoms and depressive symptoms: the role of hedonic responsivity. *Journal of Clinical Psychology*, 68(10), 1111-21. doi: 10.1002/jclp.21884.

[34] de Graaf, R., Kessler, R. C., Fayyad, J., ten Have, M., Alonso, J., Angermeyer, M., Borges, G., Demyttenaere, K., Gasquet, I., de Girolamo, G., Haro, J. M., Jin, R., Karam, E. G., Ormel, J., Posada-Villa, J. (2008). The prevalence and effects of adult attention-deficit/hyperactivity disorder (ADHD) on the performance of workers: results from the WHO World Mental Health Survey Initiative. *Occupational and Environmental Medicine*, 65(12), 835-842. doi: 10.1136/oem.2007.038448.

[35] Van den Brink, W., & Schippers, G. M., (2008). Verslaving en verslavingszorg. *Tijdschrift voor psychiatrie*, 50, 91-97 (article in Dutch).

[36] Edwards, G., & Gross, M. M. (1976). Alcohol dependence: provisional description of a clinical syndrome. *British Medical Journal*, 1(6017), 1058-1061.

[37] Li, T. K., Hewitt, B. G., Grant, B. F. (2007). The Alcohol Dependence Syndrome, 30 years later: a commentary. the 2006 H. David Archibald lecture. *Addiction,* 102(10), 1522-30.

[38] Leshner, A. I. (1997). Addiction is a brain disease, and it matters. *Science,* 3 278(5335), 45-47.

[39] McLellan, A. T., Lewis, D. C., O'Brien, C. P., Kleber, H. D. (2000). Drug dependence, a chronic medical illness: implications for treatment, insurance, and outcomes evaluation. *Journal of the American Medical Association*, 284(13), 1689-1695.

[40] Arria, A. M., & McLellan, A. T.,(2012). Evolution of concept, but not action, in addiction treatment. *Substance Use and Misuse*, 47(8-9), 1041-1048. doi: 10.3109/10826084.2012.663273.

[41] O'Brien, C. (2011). Addiction and dependence in DSM-V. *Addiction*, 106(5), 866-867. doi: 10.1111/j.1360-0443.2010.03144.x.

[42] Kendler, K. S., Chen, X., Dick, D., Maes, H., Gillespie, N., Neale, M. C., Riley, B. (2012). Recent advances in the genetic epidemiology and molecular genetics of substance use disorders. *Nature Neuroscience*, 15(2), 181-189. doi: 10.1038/nn.3018.

[43] Volkow, N. D., Fowler, J. S., Wang, G. J. (2003). The addicted human brain: insights from imaging studies. *Journal of Clinical Investigation*, 111(10), 1444–1451.

[44] Volkow, N. D., Wang, G. J., Fowler, J. S., Tomasi, D. (2012). Addiction Circuitry in the Human Brain. *Annual Review of Pharmacology and Toxicology*, 52, 321–336.

[45] Sloboda, Z., Glantz M. D., Tarter R. E. (2012). Revisiting the Concepts of Risk and Protective Factors for Understanding the Etiology and Development of Substance Use and Substance Use Disorders: Implications for Prevention. Substance Use & Misuse, 47, 944–962.

[46] Goldstein, R. Z., & Volkow, N. D. (2002). Drug addiction and its underlying neurobiological basis: neuroimaging evidence for the involvement of the frontal cortex. *American Journal of Psychiatry*, 159(10), 1642-52.

[47] Gawin, F. H., & Kleber, H. D. (1986). Abstinence symptomatology and psychiatric diagnosis in cocaine abusers: Clinical observations. *Archives of General Psychiatry*, 43, 107–113.

[48] Blum, K., Braverman, E. R., Holder, J. M., Lubar, J. F., Monastra, V. J., Miller, D., Lubar, J. O., Chen, T. J., Comings, D. E. (2000). Reward deficiency syndrome: a biogenetic model for the diagnosis and treatment of impulsive, addictive, and compulsive behaviors. *Journal of Psychoactive Drugs*, 32, 1-112.

[49] Kalechstein, A. D., Newton, T. F., Leavengood, A. H. (2002). Apathy syndrome in cocaine dependence. *Psychiatry Research*, 109, 97–100.

[50] Leventhal, A. M., Kahler, C. W., Ray, L. A., Stone, K., Young, D., Chelminski, I., & Zimmerman, M. (2008). Anhedonia and amotivation in psychiatric outpatients with fully remitted stimulant use disorder. *American Journal on Addictions*, 17, 218–223.

[51] Chandler, R. K., Fletcher, B. W., Volkow, N. D. (2009). Treating drug abuse and addiction in the criminal justice system: improving public health and safety. *Journal of the American Medical Association*, 301, 183–190.

[52] Sanfey, A.G. (2007). Social decision-making: insights from game theory and neuroscience. *Science,* 318(5850), 598–602.

[53] Glantz, M. D., & Pickens, R. W. (1992). Vulnerability to drug abuse: Introduction and overview. In M. D. Glantz, R. W. Pickens (Eds.), Vulnerability to drug abuse (pp. 1–14). Washington, D.C.: American Psychological Association.

[54] Effertz, T., & Mann, K. (2012). The burden and cost of disorders of the brain in Europe with the inclusion of harmful alcohol use and nicotine addiction. *European Neuropsychopharmacology,* 23(7), 742-748.

[55] Wittchen, H. U., Robins, L. N., Cottler, L. B., Sartorius, N., Burke, J. D., Regier, D. (1991). Cross cultural feasibility, reliability and sources of variance of the Composite International Diagnostic Interview (CIDI). The Multicentre WHO/ADAMHA Field Trials. *British Journal of Psychiatry*, 159, 645-653.

[56] van de Glind, G., Van Emmerik-van Oortmerssen, K., Carpentier, P.J., Levin, F.R., Koeter, M.W., Barta, C., Kaye, S., Skutle, A., Franck, .J, Konstenius, M., Bu, E.T., Moggi, F., Dom, G., Demetrovics, Z., Fatséas, M., Schillinger, A., Kapitány-Fövény, M., Verspreet, S, Seitz A, Johnson B, Faraone SV, Ramos-Quiroga JA, Allsop S, Carruthers S., Schoevers, R.A.; Iasp Research Group, van den Brink, W. (2013). The International ADHD in Substance Use Disorders Prevalence (IASP) study: background, methods and study population. *Int. J. Methods Psychiatr. Res.* 2013 Sep 11. doi: 10.1002/mpr.1397.

[57] Simon, V., Czobor, P., Balint, S., Meszaros, A., Bitter, I. (2009). Prevalence and correlates of adult attention-deficity hyperactivity disorder: meta-analysis. *Britisch Journal of Psychiatry,* 194(3), 204-211.

[58] Lee, S. S., Humphreys, K. L., Flory, K., Liu, R. & Glass, K. (2011). Prospective association of childhood attention-deficit/hyperactive disorder (ADHD) and substance abuse/dependence: A meta-analytic review. *Clinical Psychology Review*, 31, 328-341.

[59] Flory, K., & Lynam, D. R. (2003). The relation between attention deficit hyperactivity disorder and substance abuse: What role does conduct disorder play? *Clinical Child and Family Psychology Review*, 6, 1−16.

[60] Barkley, R. A., Fischer, M., Edelbrock, C. S., Smallish, L. (1990). The adolescent outcome of hyperactive children diagnosed by research criteria: I. An 8-year prospective follow-up study. *Journal of the American Academy of Child and Adolescent Psychiatry,* 29, 546−557.

[61] Molina, B. S., Bukstein, O. G., & Lynch, K. G. (2002). Attention-deficit/hyperactivity disorder and conduct disorder symptomatology in adolescents with alcohol use disorder. *Psychology of Addictive Behaviors*, 16,161−164.

[62] Harty, S. C., Ivanov, I., Newcorn, J. H., Halperin, J. M. (2011). The impact of conduct disorder and stimulant medication on later substance use in an ethnically diverse sample of individuals with attention-deficit/hyperactivity disorder in childhood. *Journal of Child & Adolescent Psychopharmacology*, 21(4), 331-339. doi:10.1089/cap.2010.0074.

[63] Hartsough, C. S., & Lambert, N. M. (1987). Pattern and progression of drug use among hyperactives and controls: a prospective short-term longitudinal study. *Journal of Child Psychology & Psychiatry*, 28(4), 543-553.

[64] Milberger, S., Biederman, J., Faraone, S. V., Wilens, T., Chu, M. P. (1997). Associations between ADHD and psychoactive substance use disorders. Findings from a longitudinal study of high risk siblings of ADHD children. *American Journal of Addiction*, 6(4), 318-329.

[65] Disney, E. R., Elkins, I. J., McGue, M., Iacono, W. G. (1999). Effects of ADHD, conduct disorder, and gender on substance use and abuse in adolescence. *American Journal of Psychiatry* 156(10), 1515-1521.

[66] Carpentier, P. J., van Gogh, M. T., Knapen, L. J., Buitelaar, J. K., De Jong, C. A. (2011). Influence of attention deficit hyperactivity disorder and conduct disorder on opioid dependence severity and psychiatric comorbidity in chronic methadone-

maintained patients. *European Addiction Research,* 17(1), 10-20. doi: 10.1159/000321259.

[67] Carpentier, P. J., Knapen, L. J., van Gogh, M. T., Buitelaar, J. K., De Jong, C. A. (2013). Addiction in developmental perspective: influence of conduct disorder severity, subtype, and attention deficit hyperactivity disorder on problem severity and comorbidity in adults with opioid dependence. *Journal of Addictive Disorders*, 31(1), 45-59. doi: 10.1080/10550887.2011.642756.

[68] Elkins I. J., McGue M., Iacono W. G. (2007). Prospective effects of attention-deficit/hyperactivity disorder, conduct disorder, and sex on adolescent substance use and abuse. *Archives of General Psychiatry*, 64(10), 1145-1152.

[69] Foster, I., Racicot, S., & McGrath, J. J. (2012). Attention-deficit/hyperactivity disorder subtype differentially predicts smoking expectancies in adolescents. *Journal of Adolescent Health*, 51(4), 393-9. doi: 10.1016/j.jadohealth.2012.01.014.

[70] Ivanov, I., Schultz, K. P., London, E. D., Newcorn, J. H. (2008). Inhibitory Control Deficits in Childhood and Risk for Substance Use Disorders: A Review. *The American Journal of Drug and Alcohol Abuse*, 34 (3), 239–258. doi:10.1080/00952 990802013334.

[71] Arcos-Burgos, M, Vélez J. I., Solomon, B. D., Muenke, M. (2012). A common genetic network underlies substance use disorders and disruptive or externalizing disorders. *Human Genetics*, 131(6), 917-929. doi: 10.1007/s00439-012-1164-4.

[72] Chen, K. W., Banducci, A. N., Guller, L., Macatee, R. J., Lavelle, A., Daughters, S. B., Lejuez, C. W. (2011). An examination of psychiatric comorbidities as a function of gender and substance type within an inpatient substance use treatment program. *Drug and Alcohol Dependence*, 118, 92-99.

[73] Chan, Y. F., Dennis, M. L., Funk, R. R. (2008). Prevalence and comorbidity of major internalizing and externalizing problems among adolescents and adults presenting in substance abuse treatment. *Journal of Substance Abuse Treatment*, 34(1), 14-24.

[74] Peles, E., Schreiber, S., Naumovsky, Y., Adelson, M. (2007). Depression in methadone maintenance treatment patients: rate and risk factors. *Journal of Affective Disorders ,* 99(1-3), 213-20.

[75] Compton, W. M., Cottler, L. B., Phelps, D. L., Ben Abdallah, A., Spitznagel E. L. (2000). Psychiatric disorders among drug dependent subjects: are they primary or secondary? *American Journal of Addiction*, 9(2), 126-134.

[76] Sobanski, E., Bruggemann, D., Alm, B., Kern, S., Philipsen, A., Schamalzried, H., Hesslinger, B., Waschkowski, H., Rietschel, M. (2008). Subtype differences in adults with attentiondeficit/hyperactivity disorder (ADHD) with regard to ADHD-symptoms, psychiatric comorbidity and psychosocial adjustment. *European Psychiatry*, 23(2), 142-149.

[77] Wilens, T.E., & Dodson, W. (2004). A clinical perspective of attention-deficit/hyperactivity disorder into adulthood. *Journal of Clinical Psychiatry*, 65(10), 1301-1313.

[78] Kessler, R. C., Adler, L., Barkley, R., Biederman, J., Conners, C. K., Demler, O., ..., Zaslavsky, A.M. (2006). The prevalence and correlates of adult ADHD in the United States: results from the National Comorbidity Survey Replication. *American Journal of Psychiatry,* 163, 716-723.

[79] Wilens, T. E., Tanguay. S., Chase, R., Moore, H., Faraone, S. V., Biederman, J. (2005). Characteristics of adults with attention deficit hyperactivity disorder plus substance use disorder: the role of psychiatric comorbidity. *American Journal of Addiction,* 14(4), 319-327.

[80] King V. L., Brooner R. K., Kidorf M. S., Stoller K. B., Mirsky A. F. (1999). Attention deficit hyperactivity disorder and treatment outcome in opioid abusers entering treatment. *Journal of Nervous and Mental Disease,* 187, 487–495.

[81] Levin, F. R., Evans, S. M., Kleber, H. D. (1998). Prevalence of adult attention-deficit hyperactivity disorder among cocaine abusers seeking treatment. *Drug and Alcohol Dependence,* 52, 15–25.

[82] van Emmerik-van Oortmerssen, K., van de Glind, G., Koeter, M.W., Allsop, S., Auriacombe, M., Barta, C., Bu, E.T., Burren, Y., Carpentier, P.J., Carruthers, S., Casas, M., Demetrovics, Z., Dom, G., Faraone, S.V., Fatsea, M., Franck, J., Johnson, B., Kapitány-Fövény, M., Kaye, S., Konsteniu,s M., Levin, F.R., Moggi, F., Møller, M., Ramos-Quiroga, J.A., Schillinger, A., Skutle, A., Verspreet, S.; IASP research group, van den Brink, W., Schoevers, R.A. (2014). Psychiatric comorbidity in treatment-seeking substance use disorder patients with and without attention deficit hyperactivity disorder: results of the IASP study. *Addiction.* 2014 Feb;109(2):262-72. doi: 10.1111/add.12370.

[83] Pani, P., Maremmani, I., Trogu, E., Gessa, G. L., Ruiz, P., Akiskal, H. S. (2010). Delineating the psychic structure of substance abuse and addictions: should anxiety, mood and impulse control dysregulation be included? *Journal of Affective Disorders,* 122(3), 185-197. doi: 10.1016/j.jad.2009.06.012.

[84] Bitter, I., Angyalosi, A., Czobor, P. (2012). Pharmacological treatment of adult ADHD. *Current Opinions in Psychiatry,* 25(6), 529-534. doi:10.1097/YCO.0b013e328356f87f.

[85] Fredriksen, M., Halmøy, A., Faraone, S. V., Haavik, J. (2012). Long-term efficacy and safety of treatment with stimulants and atomoxetine in adult ADHD: A review of controlled and naturalistic studies. *European Neuropsychopharmacology,* 23(6), 508-527.

[86] Faraone, S. V., & Glatt, S. J. (2010). A comparison of the efficacy of medications for adult attention-deficit/hyperactivity disorder using meta-analysis of effect sizes. *The Journal of Clinical Psychiatry,* 71(6), 754-763. doi: 10.4088/JCP.08m04902pur.

[87] Philipsen, A. (2012). Psychotherapy in adult attention deficit hyperactivity disorder: implications for treatment and research. *Expert Review of Neurotherapeutics,* 12(10), 1217-1225.

[88] Solanto, M. V., Marks, D. J., Wasserstein, J., Mitchell, K., Abikoff, H., Alvir, J. M., Kofman, M. D. (2010). Efficacy of meta-cognitive therapy for adult ADHD. *American Journal of Psychiatry,* 167(8), 958-968.

[89] Safren, S. A., Otto, M. W., Sprich, S., Winett, C. L., Wilens, T. E., & Biederman, J. (2005). Cognitive behavioral therapy for ADHD in medication-treated adults with continued symptoms. *Behaviour Research and Therapy,* 43, 831-842.

[90] National Institute for Health and Clinical Excellence (NICE). (2008). Attention deficit hyperactivity disorder. Diagnosis and management of ADHD in children, young people and adults. NICE clinical guideline 72, guidance.nice.org.uk/cg72. London: NICE.

[91] Carpentier, P. J. (2012). Addiction and the role of childhood externalizing disorders (PhD thesis). Enschede: Ipskamp Drukkers.

[92] Schubiner, H., Saules, K. K., Arfken, C. L., Johanson, C. E., Schuster, C. R., Lockhart, N., Edwards, A., Donlin, J., Pihlgren, E. (2002). Double-blind placebo-controlled trial of methylphenidate in the treatment of adult ADHD patients with comorbid cocaine dependence. *Experimental and Clinical Psychopharmacology*, 10(3), 286-294.

[93] Riggs, P. D., Hall, S. K., Mikulich-Gilbertson, S. K., Lohman, M., Kayser, A. (2004). A randomized controlled trial of pemoline for attention-deficit/hyperactivity disorder in substance-abusing adolescents. *Journal of the American Academy of Child & Adolescent Psychiatry*, 43(4), 420-429.

[94] Riggs, P. D., Winhusen, T., Davies, R. D., Leimberger, J. D., Mikulich-Gilbertson, S., Klein, C., Macdonald, M., Lohman, M., Bailey, G. L., Haynes, L., Jaffee, W. B., Haminton, N., Hodgkins, C., Whitmore, E., Trello-Rishel, K., Tamm, L., Acosta, M. C., Royer-Malvestuto, C., Subramaniam, G., Fishman, M., Holmes, B. W., Kaye, M. E., Vargo, M. A., Woody, G. E., Nunes, E. V., Liu, D. (2011). Randomized controlled trial of osmotic-release methylphenidate with cognitive-behavioral therapy in adolescents with attention-deficit/hyperactivity disorder and substance use disorders. *Journal of the American Academy of Child & Adolescent Psychiatry*, 50(9), 903-914. doi:10.1016/j.jaac.2011.06.010.

[95] Wilens, T. E., Adler, L. A., Weiss, M. D., Michelson, D., Ramsey, J. L., Moore, R. J., Renard, D., Brady, K. T., Trzepacz, P.T ., Schuh, L. M., Ahrbecker, L. M., Levine, L. R. (2008). Atomoxetine treatment of adults with ADHD and comorbid alcohol use disorders. *Drug and Alcohol Dependence*, 96(1-2), 145-154. doi: 10.1016/j.drugalcdep.2008.02.009.

[96] Levin, F. R., Evans, S. M., Brooks, D. J., Garawi, F. (2007). Treatment of cocaine dependent treatment seekers with adult ADHD: double-blind comparison of methylphenidate and placebo. *Drug and Alcohol Dependence*, 87(1), 20-29.

[97] Carpentier, P. J., de Jong, C. A., Dijkstra, B. A., Verbrugge, C. A., Krabbe, P. F. (2005). A controlled trial of methylphenidate in adults with attention deficit/hyperactivity disorder and substance use disorders. *Addiction*, 100(12), 1868-1874.

[98] Levin, F. R., Evans, S. M., Brooks, D. J., Kalbag, A. S., Garawi, F., Nunes, E. V. (2006). Treatment of methadone maintained patients with adult ADHD: double-blind comparison of methylphenidate, bupropion and placebo. *Drug and Alcohol Dependence*, 81, 137-148.

[99] Thurstone, C., Riggs, P.D., Salomonsen-Sautel, S., Mikulich-Gilbertson, C.K. (2010). Randomized, controlled trial of atomoxetine for attention-deficit/hyperactivity disorder in adolescents with substance use disorder. *Journal of the American Academy of Child & Adolescent Psychiatry*, 49(6), 573-582.

[100] Konstenius, M., Jayaram-Lindströmm , N., Beck, O., Franck, J. (2010). Sustained release methylphenidate for the treatment of ADHD in amphetamine abusers: a pilot study. *Drug and Alcohol Dependence*, 108(1-2), 130-133. doi: 10.1016/j.drugalcdep.2009.11.006.

[101] Crunelle, C. L., van den Brink, W., Veltman, D. J., van Emmerik-van Oortmerssen, K., Dom, G., Schoevers, R. A., Booij, J. (2013). Low dopamine transporter occupancy by methylphenidate as a possible reason for reduced treatment effectiveness in ADHD patients with cocaine dependence. *European Neuropsychopharmacology*. pii: S0924-977X(13)00146-6. doi: 10.1016/.

[102] Konstenius, M., Jayaram-Lindström, N., Guterstam, J., Beck, O., Philips, B., Franck, J. (2014). Methylphenidate for attention deficit hyperactivity disorder and drug relapse in criminal offenders with substance dependence: a 24-week randomized placebo-controlled trial. *Addiction*, 109(3):440-9. doi: 10.1111/add.12369.

[103] van Emmerik-van Oortmerssen, K., Vedel, E., Koeter, M.W., de Bruijn, K., Dekker, J.J., van den Brink, W., Schoevers, R.A. (2013). Investigating the efficacy of integrated cognitive behavioral therapy for adult treatment seeking substance use disorder patients with comorbid ADHD: study protocol of a randomized controlled trial. *BMC Psychiatry*. 13:132. doi: 10.1186/1471-244X-13-132.

[104] Lichtenstein, P., Halldner, L., Zetterqvist, J., Sjölander, A., Serlachius, E., Fazel, S., Långström, N., Larsson, H. (2012). Medication for attention deficit-hyperactivity disorder and criminality. *The New England Journal of Medicine*, 368(8), 776. doi: 10.1056/NEJMc1215531.

[105] van den Ban, E., Souverein, P., Meijer, W., van Engeland, H., Swaab, H., Egberts, T., Heerdink, E., (2013). Association between ADHD drug use and injuries among children and adolescents. *Eur. Child Adolesc. Psychiatry*, [Epub ahead of print].

[106] Benkert, D., Krause, K. H., Wasem, J., Aidelsburger, P., (2010). Effectiveness of pharmaceutical therapy of ADHD (Attention-Deficit/Hyperactivity Disorder) in adults - health technology assessment. *GMS Health Technol. Assess*, 6:Doc13. doi: 10.3205/hta000091.

EDITORS' CONTACT INFORMATION

Dr. Itai Berger, M.D.
Director
The Neuro-Cognitive Center
Pediatric Division
Hadassah-Hebrew University Medical Center
P.O. Box 24035, Mount Scopus
Jerusalem 91240, Israel
Tel: 972-2-584-4903
Fax: 972-2-532-8963
E-mail: itberg@hadassah.org.il

Dr. Adina Maeir, Ph.D.
Director of Cognitive Rehabilitation Track
School of Occupational Therapy Faculty of Medicine
Hadassah-Hebrew University Medical Center
School of Occupational Therapy
P.O. Box 24026, Mont Scopus
Jerusalem, Israel

INDEX

D

E

F

G

H

I

J

K

L

Q

R

S

T

U

V

W

Y